Praise for
THE RESILIENT ATHLETE

"Andrejs understands and describes very well the athletes' lifestyle and the journey that they take. This book will help anyone improve and become the best version of themselves."

—LAURA IKAUNIECE, professional track and field athlete,
WC bronze & EC silver medalist and two-time Olympian

————

"Reading *The Resilient Athlete*, I saw myself in a lot of situations and struggles that athletes go through to achieve their goals. The book shows that to reach your full potential, not only as an athlete but as a whole person, you need to live a different kind of lifestyle—a resilient lifestyle."

—ROBERTS AKMENS, professional sprint kayaker,
WC & EC medalist and Olympian

————

"A moving and insightful take on what it means to challenge your body, mind and soul in taking on an incredible endurance challenge. What I truly love about this piece is it really walks you through what putting yourself out there means."

—DAVID KILGORE, professional ultra trail runner

————

"I value Andrejs' view on being a complete athlete—where focus is placed on mental strength, complete body health and proper training approach, all without losing ambition and the fun of the sport. This book is a masterpiece and a must-read for all athletes who want to use sport as an upgrade for their live."

—HANS BRUNS, online entrepreneur and trail runner

————

T0002785

"*The Resilient Athlete* teaches us how to be "fit for life"—athletically, mentally and purposefully. The book is loaded with concepts, tools and exercises to become your best self, all "chunked" into pieces that are easy to adapt and implement."

—JEFFREY THOMAS, business investor and lifestyle athlete

"A fantastic book for the self-coached athlete! This book takes the holistic approach, giving you real world guidance on how to get smarter at training for life and sport. It's crammed with actionable points that won't just help you in your athletic endeavors—they will give you a new perspective on life!"

—RACHEL COE-O'BRIEN, physiotherapist and triathlete

"*The Resilient Athlete* is a book that I highly recommend to anyone—a seasoned athlete, a dedicated amateur, or someone trying to start their fitness journey. It has tips and tricks for you to improve your training, mentality and performance. Andrejs encourages and motivates you, no matter where you are in your journey, and shows that it is never too late to make progress."

—BETH MORGAN, white-water kayak athlete/coach and EC champion

---

"By sharing his own vulnerability and the challenges, Andrejs guides any keen athlete through a process of how to build their own solid foundation for a successful—and more importantly, enjoyable—lifetime of training. Resilience is more than just physical, and *his book* reassures us that we all have the potential and capability to harness this superpower within us."

—SYMONE GENOVEZOS, dietitian and runner

"Going way above any expectations, Andrejs has gracefully managed to pack an easy-to-read book with an extensive amount of knowledge that is summarized and broken down in a way that I know I'll be taking this book off of the bookshelf from time to time to review both mine and my students' training plans."

—KARLIS PLAKANS, adventure cyclist and fitness and calisthenics coach

---

THE
RESILIENT
ATHLETE

A SELF-COACHING GUIDE TO NEXT LEVEL PERFORMANCE IN SPORTS & LIFE

ANDREJS BIRJUKOVS

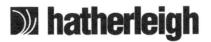

THE RESILIENT ATHLETE

Text copyright © 2023 Andrejs Birjukovs

Library of Congress Cataloging-in-Publication Data is available upon request.
ISBN: 978-1-57826-955-6

Cover and Interior Design by Carolyn Kasper

Cover Photography by Max Merget via www.fotograf-garmisch.de

Printed in the United States
10 9 8 7 6 5 4 3 2 1

CONTENTS

PREFACE

"The temptation to quit will be the greatest
just before you're about to succeed."

—CHINESE PROVERB

Nobody is immune to failure. Especially when you tread unknown waters and challenge yourself beyond what is comfortable. Which was exactly where I found myself on that unusually cold and dark August night.

It was close to sunrise and the first rays of sunlight had started to illuminate the gorgeous scenery around us. Thick green forest on the left and three-story-high red sandstone cliffs on the right. With the exception of a small campground in the place where the river makes a U-turn, the rest of the space was filled with thick reeds. Slight fog coming from the water and the sounds of nature waking up created an absolutely surreal atmosphere. On any other day, this would have been a divine experience you would go on a meditation retreat for. However, my teammate and I were not in the spirit to appreciate such beauty. Sitting on the bank of the Salaca river in rural Latvia we looked at each other—exhausted, hypothermic, hungry, and emotionally depleted.

Just half an hour ago we were on our way to win the 100-kilometer overnight kayak adventure race when our luck ran out. While covering one of the night's many river rapids we hit a boulder and ran aground. It wouldn't have been much of a problem had we used the right equipment for this adventure. A proper sea kayak as opposed to an old racing one which is much narrower and more unstable, but faster. Also, definitely, something better than a cheap head torch to illuminate the way ahead and prevent this in the first place.

Neither of us ate much throughout the night: the result of poor planning and being oblivious to what the body needs during such a long race. We were down to two fitness bars and a banana to share, all of which tasted like heaven.

Both of us were sleep-deprived and during the second half of the night I felt as though my body was moving on autopilot. The only thing that kept me in contact with reality were the floating tree branches and boulders that had a tendency to appear out of nowhere, forcing me to steer the boat at the last moment. While rapids are more technical, at least you can hear them from hundreds of meters away. Everything else floats in the water—no chance to predict or spot in complete darkness.

The worst part for me was the always present state of hypothermia. I was soaking wet and feeling cold the entire time. Even while actively kayaking, chills were going from my chest towards the fingertips. Every time we made a stop for a nature break or to grab a snack, I immediately experienced serious convulsions. My arms were shaking so badly that I had a hard time picking up and holding the paddle again.

At this point, we had covered more than two thirds of the distance, and despite running on dwindling reserves, we were determined to finish strong. That is until the universe forced us to pause and reflect. We had simply wanted to have a fun challenge at the end of the summer competition season. Instead, we found ourselves in survival mode, learning the importance of being prepared.

There it was: that fateful rapid. From afar, it looked like tens of others we had covered that night and it would not have posed an issue for a regular kayaker. However, in my sleep-deprived state, I just could not spot a clear way through: it seemed like a wall across the entire river. As we were covering it, we heard a scratching sound coming from the bottom of the boat and felt it slowing down and suddenly stopping. We ended up stuck on an underwater boulder so tight that we could not move or push ourselves in any direction. Countless minutes spent trying to break free yielded no success—the boat was stuck tight.

Everything happened in an instant. In a desperate attempt to get ourselves moving, I gave my paddle to my teammate to hold on to, stepped out waist deep in the water to lift the front of the boat and push us on a clear path. As soon as I did that, the water rushed in, filling the boat with water and tilting it to one side. The intensity of the moment made me forget about the sleep deprivation, the hunger and the hypothermia. As the strong current started pushing the boat away, I managed to hold on and jump back in at the last moment. We were moving again.

"One hell of an adventure race, isn't it?" I asked. Silence in return.

As I turned to get my paddle back, my teammate was still in shock, and I noticed that he only carried his. Turns out, once I pushed us off the boulder, he became just a passenger—the water rushed in, and he barely was able to hold on to stay in the boat and not let it float away. My paddle was taken downstream by the current. It wasn't anywhere around us, even though the morning twilight provided some visibility. The current was pushing us away quickly, so there was not much that we could do.

There we were, a pair of young, very fit, yet very inexperienced men, "stranded" on a camping spot in the middle of an adventure race that we thought we had already won. Based on our estimates, the nearest competitors were more than half an hour behind and after an intense night, we were looking forward to enjoying this last leg of the race. It was early morning, the sun started to warm the air and the route passed through a remote National Park with gorgeous views.

Instead of enjoyment, I felt frustrated, angry, and powerless, all at the same time. In the past SEVEN hours we had maneuvered down the most challenging part of the course. My teammate fell neck-deep twice in an attempt to fix a rudder broken by the underwater boulders and fallen tree branches. My legs were cramping up from having to steer and hold the rudder in a very uncomfortable position for hours.

We had expected the race to be an easy win given our background and fitness, but what we neglected in our arrogant state was the lack of experience. We did not know the terrain or how the conditions might affect the race. In some cases, we even neglected common sense. It was the night of the new moon, so it was pitch black outside. The combination of warm water and cold air created a fog and limited visibility to only 1–2 meters. And, of course, the fact that none of us had exercised for longer than three hours meant that we had no idea how our bodies would respond. We were as far out of our comfort zone as you can get.

What we relied on was that we were both athletes, competing at the highest level. Our training was hard not only physically, but also mentally. Kayaking in harsh conditions was nothing out of the ordinary for us. Training when there was snow on the ground and the splashes of water froze on the surface of the boat or 3-hour training practice was business as usual for us. However, all of that was done in a controlled environment. Most of the time we had the support of a motorboat alongside us, and safety was usually only a few minutes away. We did not realize that what we had signed up for was more serious than we expected.

There was very little talking in the few hours before the accident. We were both fighting our own demons and respected each other's need to be alone—as much as that is possible when you are in a boat together. However, sitting in an empty campground and processing what had happened, I am pretty sure that we were thinking the same thing. "There is no way we can cover 30 more kilometers with a broken rudder and just one paddle. It is just impossible." It felt as if everything was stacked against us and to this day that was the closest I have come to giving up and calling for help.

At that moment and in that miserable state we noticed a boat passing by. That meant our lead had vanished which we knew would happen eventually but witnessing it unfolding like that—with us on the sideline—felt devastating.

Taking note of our misery, the other team gave us their reserve paddle. It was for a canoe boat, so we could only use it to paddle on one side only, but it was just enough to give us hope. It would not be fast and it would not be easy, but what mattered was that all of a sudden, the impossible had become possible.

In that moment of desperation, I had an epiphany. We *had* to finish the race. No calling for help and waiting for someone to come rescue us—we'd got ourselves into this mess, and the universe was giving us an opportunity to sort it out ourselves. We had the *option* to give up, but the *opportunity* to come out stronger.

It took every ounce of our energy reserves to stay true to our goal and give it our best. On that particular day and with all the factors, our best was good enough only for 4th place. But that 4th place felt more rewarding and carries more meaning to me than a win without overcoming all that adversity. This experience pushed us to be vulnerable and accept the situation we found ourselves in. It pushed us to have the courage to remember that we started this adventure with the goal of challenging ourselves, and, of course, it pushed us to find humility and accept support.

We started the race with what we thought was a champion's mindset and were eager to win. We finished it having learned that champions are not defined by the amount or margins of their wins. Instead, they are forged by what they do when things are not working out, what standards they have for themselves, how they handle defeat, and whether they able to bounce back from failure and find their footing again.

Many years down the road we laugh and make fun of this story, remembering which one of us has gone deeper into that dark place. But one thing was clear—something had shifted in me and I felt that shift was permanent. We had the opportunity to give up and call for help, but something inside hesitated to do that. Something inside us did not want to accept things to end if it did not do so on our terms.

This was the first time I felt what resilience was in practice.

INTRODUCTION: HERO'S JOURNEY

What separates a champion from any other athlete?

While the obvious answer would be the gold medal, whoever wins the race is crowned the champion, but that is not the whole story. Sure, it's impressive to witness someone delivering top performance, but why are we then sometimes left unimpressed by "easy" wins?

Results alone do not make someone an inspiring figure, and top performance does not automatically qualify an athlete to become a role model for true sportsmanship. Such a status is deeply rooted in perseverance and grit. We need our champions to earn glory the hard way: to go through hardships, fight for it, be on the verge of losing it all only to bounce back stronger. Such adversity makes the journey relatable and is also the essence of the Olympic dream. Often, individual stories of the struggles that athletes go through to qualify for and get to the Olympic Games are more captivating and inspiring than the competition itself.

It is purpose and vision which drive athletes to put in the training hours. Faith and perseverance to recover from injuries and setbacks. Courage to get on the starting line and face the competition. Unwillingness to give up on themselves. Whatever the obstacles, these are the character traits that symbolize sportsmanship, grab our attention, and earn champions their respect. In this realm, one can become a champion without earning a gold medal. They become champions in their own class.

It is called the Hero's Journey,[1] an alluring narrative pattern that describes a person (hero) venturing into the unknown. He or she is faced with many challenges and obstacles

---

1   Coined by Joseph Campbell in his book *The Hero with a Thousand Faces*, the Hero's Journey is a 12-step framework used to create a compelling narrative based on myths and stories from a broad range of cultures.

throughout the quest, but nonetheless returns home victorious and transformed. Sounds captivating, doesn't it?

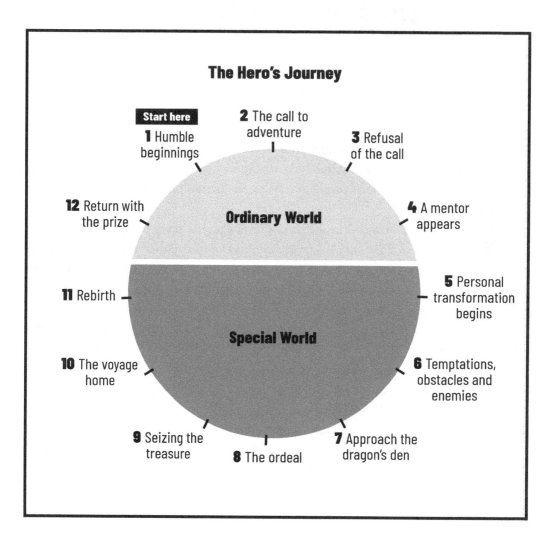

12 Stages of the Hero's Journey. Figure created in reference to Joseph Campbell's book, The Hero with a Thousand Faces.

We often hear and read these stories of personal transformation or physical triumph. "Man loses over 250 pounds and completes a marathon. 56-year-old swims across the Atlantic Ocean. Man with Down Syndrome completes Ironman triathlon." Mostly these are the stories of the so-called underdogs—people who at the first glance seem to have little chance for success—performing against all odds. It's also a recurring theme that is promoted by social media—the everyman meets unforeseen obstacles, back against the wall and odds stacked against him or her, compelled to seek strength deep within. Rather than abandon the journey or surrendering in the face of adversity, he or she finds purpose and that experience to become more self-actualized and thus, resilient.

There is something universal and very powerful in such heroic stories, and we all connect with them on an emotional level. **Each of us is on our own Hero's Journey to our own personal triumph**—be it running a marathon, trekking in the Himalayas, learning to surf, or simply playing football with our children. Very often on this quest, we are looking for a guide, a mentor or a role model that has found success before and can show us the path.

Champions, role models or heroes, call them whatever you wish, are first and foremost resilient athletes. They are not only physically fit, but also able to deliver when it matters, to accumulate their skills, training and motivation, and to unleash it all at that one moment when the pressure is high. Consistently, despite the setbacks.

Resilient athletes are able to routinely deliver top performance because they set themselves up for it throughout the years. They are made of all the days and things we do not see and not just by hard physical training. It is also the small daily practices that shape character, patience, discipline, focus, good habits, early mornings, personal sacrifices, overcoming doubt, fear, and much more.

Resilient athletes give their best when nobody's watching and have faith when nobody believes in them. They are in the game for the long term—not just a season or two. Resilient athletes treat their fitness as an extension of their identity, instead of it being a means to earn a medal.

Resilient athletes build themselves from the ground up to have an ultimate life experience—to be able to weather the storms of life, to accept uncertainty and to understand that things may not go their way. And when things do go wrong, they are able to pick themselves up and keep going.

At its core, resilience is the muscle that helps us get back up every time the world knocks us to our knees. It is a driving force that moves us forward and guides us when we choose faith over fear. It helps us tackle anything head on and overcome any setback that we might face. It reminds us that at our core we are more than anything we will ever face. Much like any muscle, resilience requires training through practice. The experiences that athletes have throughout their careers strengthen that muscle. Not only the thrills of racing and adventure, but also the back-office activities, like pushing through the pain, handling defeat, recovering from injuries, controlling emotions, and constantly reinventing yourself to become better, faster and stronger.

We look up to our role models, because ultimately, we want to build similar resilience and use it in our own lives. Do not stay injured, frustrated with lack of progress, overtrained, or burned out, like many amateur and self-coached athletes do. Develop the ability to quiet down the noise of everyday life, focus immensely and perform despite the pressure.

In reality, life's greatest journey is not running 100 meters in under 10 seconds, rowing across the Atlantic Ocean, or even running seven marathons on seven continents in seven days. It is not about finding the next big challenge or a whirlwind adventure to embark on. **Life's greatest journey is about making peace with yourself and living the complete experience every day.** One that is balanced between the internal world of fitness, skills, capabilities and purpose, and the external world of events, connections, and uncertainty. What is the purpose of physical triumph, if it comes at the expense of success in other areas of your life?

I have been there myself—chasing peak fitness and struggling on a journey to what I thought was optimal athletic performance. Trying to get to the next level, but with limited knowledge of what to do, repeating the same thing over and over again. In my combined 20+ years of competitive kayaking, running and triathlon experience, I have done it all. I have won races and finished in the second half of the pack. I have felt on top of the world and suffered from fatigue, mental and physical burnout. I have been overtrained or injured and forced to start from the beginning. Lacked time to exercise and struggled with getting results despite putting in many hours of training.

On one particular occasion, during a mid-season performance testing at the laboratory, I found myself exactly where I had been at the start of the season. My aerobic and anaerobic thresholds had not improved despite months of hard workouts and pushing myself to the limits. Something was not right, and a lot was about to change.

I turned to my role models for answers, ideas, and secrets only to realize that most successful athletes are the ones who make training their lifestyle. They incorporate it into daily life and tweak all things impacting performance until they find the recipe that works for them. It was a massive undertaking to re-think my entire lifestyle, but the idea of building myself up to the point of being unbreakable (the word I used in my mind) was very appealing to me. This did not necessarily mean getting better at racing, but to become stronger for life, to befriend the discomfort and handle harder challenges. I wanted to make myself strong all around—mentally and physically—to weather any storm of life.

Fast forward a few years later, I have embraced the self-coaching approach and started to organize my lifestyle differently one small step at a time. While I was still training with the team, I was doing so on my own terms, writing most of my training programs myself, listening to my body, adjusting the workload to fit my condition and paying attention to areas I had overlooked earlier. For example, recovery, nutrition and lifestyle habits. That was when things finally started to shift big time. All metrics were up—VO_2max, thresholds, overall endurance, strength, peak power, and, more importantly, I started to feel unbreakable.

For a long time, I lived in search of peak performance. I was stuck in tunnel vision focused on a specific race/result, looking to squeeze out every ounce of energy I have, only to arrive at the finish line with nothing left to give. In a weird way, exhausting myself fully brought a sense of achievement and made me feel good about myself, like it meant that I had given it my best shot. However, what I have found for myself, and consistently notice in the athletes that I coach, is that while peaks come and go, life goes on. **The excitement of achieving something might last for a day, a week, or a few months, but it eventually fades because the peak is never the end destination.**

What looks like a mountain to climb at first glance is just one milestone on a longer journey, kind of like a stepping stone to a new height—a bigger vision. Not necessarily in a linear way (i.e., running faster or lifting more weight), but rather a new height in life. That's another thing that makes someone feel good about themselves—making progress. Expanding horizons, pushing the boundaries of what is possible, and living on your own terms. Just like athletes peak for their key races, we go through intense periods when we work towards a certain goal. Even if we do not know it when we start, there is always a better view once we reach the top and always a new destination that we end up going to.

Resilient athletes do not put their entire lives on hold to zero in on one specific race or challenge. Instead, they understand the long-term value of self-care and creating foundational strength in their body and mind. They are in it for the long haul and build themselves from the ground up to withstand any pressure, are able to jump on any opportunity, and take any challenge life throws at them. **Becoming resilient is not an overnight thing, but a continuous process.** On this quest, every day and every effort to do the right thing (instead of taking a shortcut) counts.

This book is a step-by-step framework designed to build foundational fitness and develop resilience through a gradual mindset and lifestyle changes. On the pages that follow, you will find actionable advice to incorporate into your daily life one small step at a time. It includes strategies to cultivate the mindset to overcome setbacks and grow in confidence, and systems to adopt healthy lifestyle habits to have more energy and feel less stressed. And, of course, training tactics to get fit for all those experiences and adventures you dream of having throughout your lifetime.

This book is essentially a series of self-coaching sessions that are not geared towards one particular sport, but rather focus on creating an ultimate athletic experience—one where physical and emotional states are in balance with purpose.

The layout of the book is split into three parts: mindset, lifestyle, and training. This breakdown helps to dissect the idea of a resilient athlete into easy-to-understand bits. One thing to remember is that these three parts are inter-connected and need to be considered as a whole to really work. The lifestyle will not be sustainable if even one of the areas is out of balance. For example, being fit and strong might be the most desired aspect of being an athlete, but without a healthy lifestyle to balance it out, athletes won't be able to sustain the workload (injuries, poor recovery, lack of energy, excuses, work commitments and so on). On the other hand, when someone trains with no purpose (beyond losing some weight or growing some muscles), then he/she faces a risk of stagnating or not being consistent enough to see tangible results.

If you feel stuck on your journey to optimal health and fitness, then my advice is to keep going. Regardless of whether you are just getting started or are an experienced athlete feeling far removed from your athletic past, this book will bring coaching techniques into your own hands and will empower you to take control of your life. The tactics I share will not only get you to your next peak (whatever that is for you) but will help you achieve long-term sustainability as an athlete.

I wish you all success in your own Hero's Journey and am more than happy to share it with you!

PART I

Mindset

AM I RESILIENT OR NOT?

If asked to reflect, how would you rate your life right now? Are you a 10 out of 10 beyond excited about where things are headed? Or do you feel more like a five or a six, looking to make a change for the better? Either way, what would you use as a measurement tool? Is it the variety of skills you possess, depth of relationships, the way you look/feel, things you own, results achieved, your contribution to society, or all of the above?

Instead, how about measuring the quality of our lives by the caliber of experiences we get to have?

Some experiences will be joyous and uplifting moments. As athletes, we are no strangers to being thrilled and excited by events and adventures or fulfilled by achievements. We live for those butterflies we feel in our stomach a minute before the gun goes off. We seek the endorphins that are released the second we cross the finish line of our first marathon (and think "never again"). And we crave the excitement that precedes taking those first steps of the Everest Base Camp Trek.

But there's the other side as well. And more often than not we tend to remember the tougher periods of life as our formative years. Challenging situations we have gone through, setbacks and pressure we have faced, or even losses we have experienced. Even though there is little fun in dealing with pain and struggle, such obstacles are the mechanism for advancing further in life. It's like building muscle—growth requires resistance, so whoever is ready to go through pain and discomfort will emerge stronger on the other side.

Success in sports is often seen as very physical, be faster, stronger, jump higher, but after a certain point, it becomes increasingly mental. The way that an athlete trains and competes always reflects what happens inside his or her head. If an athlete loses or struggles in training, very often he or she faces difficulties in other areas of life as well. For example, relationship issues, a stressful job, fatigue, etc. When an athlete succeeds, be it winning, setting a personal record, or coming back from injury, he or she triumphs over fears and doubts, displaying courage in the face of adversity. In fact, in most professional sports, the competition is so high that the difference between the winner and the runner up is hardly visible. The gold medal and confetti usually go to whoever wants it the most, is able to embrace the pain and discomfort for longer and does not give up until the end.

All of that adversity isn't only there to make our lives harder. Whatever we go through in life is invested into a virtual bank account and becomes, sort of, an "experience fund" that we live off later in life. Dealing with setbacks helps us adapt to harder challenges, learn to carry on when things get bumpy and resist the temptation to quit. It is thanks to those low points of our journey that we become who we are, grow into a more resilient person, and are able to fully enjoy peak experiences.

Looking at some of the most inspiring athletes of the modern age, like Michael Phelps (swimming), Eliud Kipchoge (marathon running), Lindsey Vonn (alpine skiing), Usain Bolt (100m sprint), Serena Williams (tennis), Cristiano Ronaldo (soccer), Bethany Hamilton (surfing), and Craig Alexander (iron-distance triathlon) one thing is certain, they have all been in the spotlight for a while. It was not smooth sailing for any of them because staying at the top of your game requires a lot of conscious effort to constantly reinvent yourself and deal with unexpected setbacks (injuries, defeat, stress of daily life). This consistency throughout many years, staying true to your purpose, and delivering when the pressure is high is a mark of a resilient athlete.

In its essence, resilience is the ability of an object to bounce back into shape when deformed. **Or, to put it into a different perspective, being able to stand back up when life has brought you down—to recover from difficulties.**

It is easy to do the right thing when everything is set up for that, to train hard when fully recovered and healthy, eat a nutritious diet when everything is prepared, sleep 8+ hours when there is no need to juggle two different jobs, or to stay calm in a monastery somewhere high in the Himalayas. Being resilient is about doing the right thing even when everything is against you, having faith, and giving your best in times of stress, adversity and uncertainty. For instance, when an injury forces an athlete to stop training, being resilient means having the courage to let go of expectations and start from the beginning. When there is a lot of pressure or stress in life, being resilient means re-thinking your schedule to allow more down time to come back recharged and stronger. When an athlete approaches the end of his career, being resilient means not stopping the training process just because there is no racing. Instead, continue to exercise because it has become part of the lifestyle and identity.

Resilience is always about the long-term. It's a combination of factors and experiences that we face throughout our life that keeps us going. A product of focus, determination, discipline, willpower and, of course, habits, it is the driving force that allows an athlete to function at the top level and consistently deliver his best, whatever that might be on a particular day.

So, what drives someone to push through the hard moments and simply refuse to quit, neither in a race nor in life? What's the secret sauce that allows an athlete to show up every day, put in the work and to progress over the years? To answer that and understand how to become a resilient athlete, we need to look closer at what it actually means.

MENTAL TOUGHNESS

A lot about peak performance has to do with conditioning the mindset and being able to distance yourself from the situation and distractions. Showing up prepared is only the first step to being able to go through a hard challenge or a long-distance race. In order to show what you are truly capable of you have to be able to let go of expectations, concerns and doubts, so that you can anchor yourself in the present moment, focus on how you feel and what you need to do right now.

Elite athletes are particularly good at focusing immensely on the task at hand to quiet down the noise of the outside world (or negative thoughts in the head) and deliver top performance when the pressure is high. That process of blocking out everything else is what we see on TV when an athlete puts on his or her headphones and makes a poker face to quiet down the chatter and reach deep within to remember all of the training they have done to get to that moment. It is very hard to do, but years of practice in training and competing make it look like second nature.

Splitting a large task into smaller chunks and focusing on the very next step is a well-known productivity hack, but it also helps us to focus better and reduce the overall pressure that comes with going beyond the comfort zone.

Sometimes called mental toughness, such focus is the basis for having the discipline to be consistent in training, give your best during a race and do what seems impossible for the rest of the world. For some people, it comes naturally, while others (Michael Phelps included) need to work hard to develop the skill.

FOCUS AND VISUALIZATION: MICHAEL PHELPS AT THE BEIJING OLYMPICS

In one of his interviews Michael Phelps's coach Bob Bowman shared how Michael had a hard time managing his attention and energy early on in his swimming career. He was unable to focus in class and was easily distracted. Some teachers even raised concerns to his mom, Debbie, that her son would not achieve much in life. However, after many years of consistent relaxation and visualization practice every night, he built a skill that helped him stay focused and confident under tremendous pressure.

In fact, his focusing technique is one of the key factors that earned him eight gold medals in a single week during the Beijing Olympics. And one race in that competition stands out the most—the 200-meter butterfly final. As soon as he dove in his goggles broke and started to fill in with water. He continued on, despite the situation becoming worse with every stroke. After the last turn and with 50 meters left to go Phelps was barely ahead of his nearest competitor and just under the world record. He had only to finish strong—something he's the best in the world at—but by this time his goggles were completely filled with water leaving him absolutely blind. No opportunity to tell how far the finish is and where the competition is.

In his daily practice he envisioned the entire race, start to finish. He went through every stroke and knew how many he needed on every length of the pool to get from one wall to another. So, instead of panicking, he played a mental video of the race in his head and relied on that vision to bring him home. He made the last stroke and reached for the wall hoping it would be there and hoping he wouldn't smash into it with his head—earning his 10th gold medal and breaking the world record by 0.06 of a second.

It is unbelievable how, at the most elite level of competition, Michael has overcome a setback that probably would have undermined most other swimmers' confidence. When the pressure was on and it was time to perform, he could literally do it with his eyes closed. He already envisioned the race in his head, so when the obstacle appeared he knew he could deliver. If you watch the replay, you cannot even tell there's a problem—the stroke is smooth and rhythmic, just as in any other race.

The good news is that anyone can develop such skills. It is not that some people are missing a setting in the brain that's called "grit, willpower, and perseverance." With the right techniques we can influence our beliefs, abandon those that do not serve us and build new more empowering ones. Each of us can control the way we respond to certain emotions and, as a result, handle ourselves in times of stress.

The phrase "mental toughness" can be misleading because it implies that an athlete should be "tough" and show no vulnerability. Hiding emotions, putting on a brave face no matter what to keep the world from knowing what you are going through is a surefire way to an emotional burnout. Ignoring emotions makes them pile up and as the time passes it gets increasingly harder to self-regulate and process what happens inside the head, which, in turn, impacts focus, energy and drive. A sustainable way of building long-term resilience is to take the time to rest, reflect, understand emotions, and learn to deal with them.

Fear, doubt, concern, anxiety, the more we face and understand what drives these emotions instead of hiding them the more we condition ourselves to know our worth, look at the positive, focus on ourselves and have the courage to be imperfect. This focus trains our minds to self-regulate in times of stress, stay calm under pressure, and become what they call more mentally and emotionally strong. That is what allows us to make the leap and reach for the stars, to resist that small demon, elf, gnome or whoever sits on our shoulder asking Are you sure you can do it? Are you sure you are worthy?

PHYSICAL WELL-BEING

A lot of the athletes are type A personalities, so when there is an obstacle, their first response is to push through and overcome it, against all odds. Turn on the gladiator mode and carry on, as if it is business as usual. Such a mindset is indeed very powerful in overcoming challenges, pushing yourself to the limits, and delivering top performance. However, it can also be a trap that many athletes fall into.

Competitiveness on a daily basis, testing yourself on every workout, increasing volume without careful planning or not recognizing the difference between healthy and unhealthy pain, has a risk of obscuring the athlete's vision. Ambitions have a tendency to blind people to the point where they might make a decision in favor of short-term performance over longevity in the sport. For example, if the setback you are faced with is injury or sickness, then it is not helpful to train through it hoping the pain will pass on its own. A better strategy would be to take time off, fully recover, and use the opportunity to work on weak areas to build yourself up even stronger.

Living in a competitive mindset does not work long-term. It is not always a race against the clock or an effort to overcome fear and doubt, or even a need to push beyond limits to prove something. Performance is not only about what we condition our mind to focus on, but also what our physical bodies are able to support. Often athletes set very high goals and expect to reach them in a very short timeframe by placing a lot of training load on their bodies. However, sometimes despite our ambitions we have to swallow our ego and focus on what is best for our body at the moment and in the long term.

The process of building a high level of fitness that will support you throughout your entire life is slow and incremental. There's a limit to how much we can push our bodies without taxing physical and psychological systems to the point of burnout. This is why it takes many years for athletes to reach world-class levels of performance (and some never do). It is a process of building, recovering and repeating that spans across multiple years. There is a lot of nuance that goes into developing an athlete and everything needs to be balanced to work seamlessly—mobility, strength, aerobic engine, power, speed, agility, skills, etc.

This need for balance is why an athlete's health is the only thing that matters. Without it, we can only dream of all the great things we could do if we were healthy or were not injured. Top level athletes do everything in their power to protect their health and avoid days of being forced not to train. They do not just train to get stronger but consider what is best for the body. In particular, which lifestyle habits stimulate good performance, and which undermine it. How does diet affect health and performance? How can you prevent or treat any medical condition that might affect longevity in the sport? The reason athletes are such perfectionists about their daily habits is found in the quote by Will Durant "We are what we repeatedly do. Excellence, then, is not an act, but a habit." Over time small habits build up, creating a strong and healthy foundation with which come more energy and drive.

A physically resilient person is someone who is able to stick to the habits and routines that support physical health and fight off any diseases or injuries.

PERSONAL ATTRIBUTES

Looking at our individual Heroes' Journeys, it is not enough to push through the obstacles and be strong and healthy to deliver great results. We also need to have a personality and courage to walk our own path.

It might feel rewarding to be completely exhausted after finishing a hard workout or running a marathon. But after some time, maybe a few races or even a few years, the question inevitably comes. It might happen that you ask it yourself at a particularly vulnerable time or someone (friends or family) does that for you. *What's next? Why am I doing this?* If you do not have a confident answer to that, you risk getting "stuck" or even abandoning the journey altogether. After not getting expected results, some athletes might start feeling they are not enough or not worthy or even a "failure." Such thoughts can easily be amplified by social media which tends to showcase only the best parts of life and lead to the belief that others' lives are so fulfilling and free of problems.

We need a purpose behind our actions to be able to carry the motivation all the way through. A vision of why we started in the first place which will serve as a heading for us to stick to.

The good feeling of exhausting yourself might come from doing a good job and making progress towards better fitness, but at some point, that excitement wanes. Every athlete should answer for themselves the question of what lies beyond workouts and competitions.

For what purpose is this pursuit of fitness? Is it worth making sacrifices for? Answers to these questions will help you to determine whether the lifestyle and fitness are sustainable in the long term, far beyond a competitive career. Having a purpose that is bigger than any particular workout or a race makes a person feel that he or she advances in life, comes closer to achieving lifetime goals/dreams, or contributes to other people's lives.

The Japanese call it *ikigai*—something that gives a person a sense of purpose or a reason for living. It is a combination of things you are good at, things you love, things the world needs and things you can be paid for. However, a purpose is not something that is expected of us or otherwise external. To have the power to propel us forward, our purpose has to be generated from within by focusing on our own lives.

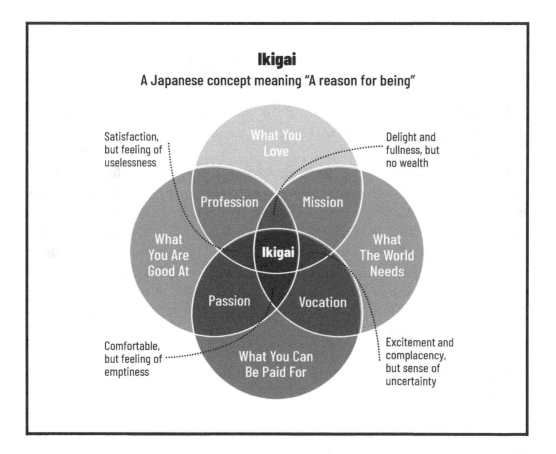

Illustration based on the framework presented in the book Ikigai: The Japanese Secret to a Long and Happy Life, *written by Héctor García.*

Unfortunately, we live in a world dominated by opinions, advertisement, and peer pressure. Sometimes the external message is so "loud" that individuals are often pushed to accept things they are not passionate about. Knowing who we are, what we stand for and owning it takes confidence. Which is why besides purpose, personality is also formed by values, standards, degrees of self-awareness, and even skills we possess. They say we do not rise to the occasion, but rather fall to the level of preparation and an athlete, like any person, needs to carry a vast arsenal of skills, capabilities, values and standards to be resilient and ready to tackle any obstacles before they even appear.

THE EXTERNAL WORLD

Imagine a very fit and determined individual en route to ascent mount Everest. He or she has trained for well over a year and is well-equipped to reach the summit of the world's tallest mountain. That person has a strong purpose behind the ordeal (maybe even doing it for charity) and is eager to raise the flag of home country while standing at the top of the world. What is so special about this, you ask? That individual would be doing the entire adventure completely alone. Yes, trekking to the base camp, carrying provisions, acclimatizing, cooking food, establishing tents and safety ropes, navigating the weather and terrain, and essentially spending a few months in solitude. How much of a chance for success would you give that person?

Hard to imagine, right? That's because as much as it might feel very "macho" to go at it alone, rely on yourself, succeed on your own terms and prove something, is a very ego-driven approach, and very ineffective. The result of the team's work will always be better and more significant than that of an individual. Joining an organized expedition or at least hiring a group of people to help carry the load and partner with other climbers would offer a much better chance of success (and survival). The same goes for life and sport. We are not expected to do everything alone. Besides, everything that's worth fighting for is best shared, which is why we need a team, a coach, or at least a mentor on our journey to assist us.

"If you want to go fast, go alone. If you want to go far, go together."

— AFRICAN PROVERB

The way we interact with the external world sets us up for an ultimate experience. Life is not about locking yourself up in the monastery to practice self-awareness and regulation, perfect physique, and skills, as well as find inner peace. No, it is those connections and support networks (teams, coaches and mentors) that we create, new and unusual things we try, and the uncertainty that we embrace is what challenges us. All of that challenge and the external factors help us to understand ourselves better and find ways to improve.

Practice does make perfect, but change is a significant aspect that helps develop resilience. We live in patterns, go to the same grocery store, do the same workouts, same routines. Life is optimized and, as my father often jokes, "the body strives for simplicity and the least energy expenditure." This is true, but what it also entails is that on a daily basis we do not experience the pain or discomfort to which our body can adapt and ultimately grow.

Back when I was a professional kayaker, I remember wishing for conditions to be easier. For some competitors not to participate, for the wind not to blow hard, or for the waves to be smaller and less bumpy. Actually, for everything to line up flawlessly, so that I could execute my perfect race. However, after transitioning to triathlons where a lot of things can go wrong in a single race, I realized how silly it was of me to rely on external conditions. In that mindset, I was essentially a prisoner, because I was questioning my performance and confidence. After all, conditions were the same for everybody and not everything can be perfect every time. So, the healthiest approach is to learn to live with it and be ready to execute in any conditions. Instead of wishing for things to be easy, wish to be stronger and able to withstand anything.

Magic starts to happen when we start exposing ourselves to new ideas, training methods, people, and even external factors. Once we take that leap to do something new and uncomfortable, we are less afraid of repeating it the next time. **It is always the first step that's terrifying, but when we push out of our comfort zone like this, it shifts a little further with each small effort.**

In exercise physiology, this principle is called progressive overload. Athletes gradually increase the duration, frequency, and intensity of the exercise with the purpose of adapting the body to a higher workload. Eventually, what felt hard or uncomfortable earlier becomes the new normal. This principle works for the physical body as much as it does for the mind. Explore a new route on your next bike or run session, instead of the one you know by heart. You might get lost and frustrated about it, but that is part of the process. A great way to challenge existing beliefs about your current fitness is to try a new sport altogether and, who knows, maybe it will spark a new passion.

By putting ourselves in different situations and facing external factors, we let our mind get used to the idea that we are not in control of many things and that's OK. It is important to accept this fact because it helps to widen your perspective and be open to new (and maybe more exciting) experiences. When things do go wrong and the pressure is on, the mind will be conditioned to deliver in spite of that.

THE RESILIENT ATHLETE

As athletes, self-confidence is our thing. We tend to have little doubt that we will find a way to achieve whatever we put our mind to. The question is always how fast we can do it and the big challenge so many of us face is finding balance on the way to those goals.

For example, spending more time on quality training will make an athlete fitter, but not everyone has that extra time and attention to spare every day. Moreover, it is not enough to be physically fit and disciplined to handle life's challenges or able to recover from setbacks.

The resilient athlete is someone who balances purposeful training with a healthy lifestyle and recognizes that having this balance is paramount to being confident, prepared to weather the storms of life and deliver when the pressure is high. Not once and not only on race day—overall.

This might seem like a very vague subject. After all, what one considers a triumph over setbacks might be business as usual for another because resilience has four different angles (domains) to consider: character strengths, emotional well-being and regulation, physical health, and the external world.

Each individual will resonate with and place more value on the domain that overcomes the type of adversity which he or she is facing at the moment. For example, athletes who struggle to calm themselves down in a moment of stress may be inspired by those who won't bend under pressure. Those who cannot seem to start exercising consistently may wonder what drives others to show up every day without fail.

Character strengths

- Vision/purpose
- Personal standards
- Work ethic and consistency
- Growth mindset
- Humor, optimism, and faith

Emotional well-being and regulation

- Self-awareness
- Emotional regulation
- Ability to focus
- Unwillingness to give up
- Empowering beliefs

External world

- Support system (coaches, mentors)
- Team/community
- Social connectedness
- Resistance to environmental/ other factors

Physical health

- Physical attributes (strength, endurance, mobility, etc.)
- Diet and lifestyle habits
- Absence of injuries/medical conditions
- Longevity in sport

Resilience domains and their manifestation.

Many athletes fall into a trap of trying to oversimplify their training and focus on the one thing that they believe is the key to add more volume, improve strength, include certain speed intervals, reduce fat percentage, or even improve lung capacity. While each individual aspect does impact performance, such isolation puts a limit on the long-term progress they can achieve and will eventually lead to plateau, stagnation and, as a result, frustration. Being good at any sport requires a mix of different capabilities—physical (i.e., strength, speed, endurance), lifestyle (i.e., recovery, diet, habits) and mindset (i.e., work ethic, purpose, standards).

When an athlete blends these four domains in a balanced way, he or she becomes a resilient athlete. Not necessarily an athlete who looks to improve one specific attribute to a maximum while putting the rest on hold. Instead, optimize a lot of small things that over time add up. This approach helps to create a lifestyle around sport so we can stay in the game for longer, and more importantly, enjoy it.

Resilient athletes show up when nobody is watching because there is a deep purpose behind training, not a desire to impress others. They welcome change and embrace pain, discomfort and the unknown, because that is the only way to grow. They refuse to quit even when odds are stacked against them because it is not about the result, but rather who they become in the process. Resilient athletes build themselves up not to reach a peak, but to have strength to traverse it towards an even bigger mountain ahead.

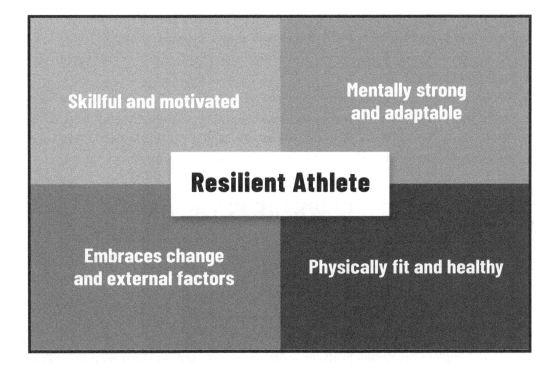

Attributes of a resilient athlete based on four resilience domains.

So, where do you go from here?

When the world, especially social media, is obsessed with attention, overnight success, instant fame and so on, it might be tempting to take a leap of faith and make a radical life change. However, these changes always take time and are usually pretty intimidating to begin with, which is why the practice of building resilience starts with overcoming small obstacles on a daily basis. Small wins and consistent lifestyle shifts end up having a huge long-term impact and often are even more powerful than big, I-am-a-new-person ones. Why? Because small actions are more sustainable, and they accumulate over time. Just like driving a train, if you want to turn it, you need to do it gradually. Making small lifestyle adjustments is like turning the tracks by a few inches and over time until you find yourself in a completely different destination than you were headed to originally.

The progress we make in life will be determined by how much conscious effort we put into working on ourselves, but before beginning anything (a training program or a transformation journey) we need to establish a starting point. No matter how accomplished an athlete or how happy you are as a person, there are always areas that could use some focus. We all have those, even the greatest athletes acknowledge a gap between where they are and where they want to be.

Use the questions ahead to take a "helicopter" view of your life and discover where you excel and what areas you can improve in to become more resilient. Identify what really matters to you and use that as a focus throughout this book. With any of the tactics shared ahead, think of an end result and visualize it materializing.

EXERCISE: WHERE IS THE GAP?

The following exercise will help you categorize your life into four resilience domains, so that you can identify specific areas that are currently "out of balance" and need improvements. More often than not, it is these very areas which are causing the most amount of stress and frustration and obstruct the path to becoming a better athlete.

As you go through the questions remember that no athlete is perfect and it is impossible to achieve complete satisfaction in all areas. Part of the pressure of being a high achiever is that we always strive for perfection. However, a great athlete is a well-rounded one and by learning about ourselves, we can find weak points and use relevant strategies to improve them one at a time.

Consider each domain like a spoke in a wheel. When one is shorter than the rest, handling the entire bike becomes very challenging. The same concept applies to our lives, when the balance is skewed towards one of the four domains, we tend to avoid challenges that are not associated with that. For example, someone who is physically fit but finds it hard to control their emotions might try to avoid or be anxious about high-pressure situations or interactions. As a result, he or she will either underperform or avoid the opportunity altogether.

To answer the question whether you are resilient or not, rate each of the questions below on a scale from 1 to 10. Be totally honest with yourself—there's nobody to judge you. Your total for the domain will be the average of the group.

CHARACTER STRENGTHS	SCORE
How fulfilled are you with the way in which you are currently living your life? *(1 = not at all fulfilled, 10 = totally fulfilled)*	
How much do you look forward to the day ahead every morning? *(1 = not looking forward at all, 10 = very much looking forward)*	
Are you confident and secure in who you are as a person? *(1 = not at all confident, 10 = totally confident)*	
How much easier would your life be if you were more disciplined? *(1 = a lot easier, 10 = not much different)*	
How strongly do you feel about your purpose? *(1 = I don't have one, 10 = I'm passionate about my purpose)*	
Average score	
EMOTIONAL WELL-BEING AND REGULATION	SCORE
How mentally healthy (and strong) do you currently feel? *(1 = not at all healthy, 10 = totally healthy)*	
To which extent can you handle a high-pressure situation and remain calm? *(1 = I'm not good at all, 10 = I'm very confident and calm)*	
How able are you to refrain from retaliation (i.e., if someone is rude/provocative) *(1 = I can't control myself, 10 = I can refrain easily)*	
How often negative emotions (i.e., anger, anxiety, guilt) get the "better" of you? *(1 = constantly, 10 = never)*	
Are you impacted easily on an emotional level? *(1 = I'm impacted very easily, 10 = I'm not impacted at all)*	
Average score	

PHYSICAL HEALTH	SCORE
How happy are you about your current physical health/fitness? *(1 = not at all satisfied, 10 = extremely happy)*	
How active are you throughout the day/week? *(1 = I don't move unless I have to, 10 = I don't sit still)*	
How energized do you feel throughout the entire day? *(1 = I'm always drained, 10 = I have more energy than I can spend)*	
How would you rate the quality of your diet (including snacks and eating out)? *(1 = terrible, 10 = 100% healthy)*	
How would you rate the quality of your sleep? *(1 = I feel drained every morning, 10 = I feel totally recharged every morning)*	
Average score	

EXTERNAL FACTORS	SCORE
How happy are you with the overall quality of your relationships? *(1 = very unsatisfied, 10 = very happy)*	
How much do you encourage and support those closest to you? *(1 = don't encourage at all, 10 = I'm the best cheerleader)*	
How open are you to accepting feedback and changing your approach? *(1 = I always know better, 10 = I'm always open to change)*	
How consistent are you in stepping out of your comfort zone and taking new risks? *(1 = I love comfort, 10 = I consistently step into the unknown)*	
To what extent external factors and uncertainty can derail you? *(1 = I depend on external factors, 10 = make my own fortune)*	
Average score	

Which of the domains you scored the least in? Was it the one you felt was falling behind or have you discovered more about yourself? Either way, the questions below will help you dig deeper and guide you to discover how to take control of those areas. Notice that the questions turn the table to you and focus on what you can do about the situation.

RESILIENCE DOMAIN	QUESTIONS FOR SELF-REFLECTION
Character Strengths	• What am I good at? • Who are my role models and what do I like about them? • How would I describe my ideal self? • What beliefs are holding me from becoming that person? • What traits, attitudes, skills, abilities, and beliefs do I need to develop to become that person?
Emotional Well-Being and Regulation	• When do I feel on top of the world? • On what occasions do I doubt myself or think *"what if?"* • Which events or situations trigger negative emotions (anger, anxiety, fear, etc.)? • How can I navigate those situations better? • What can I do to feel on top of the world every day?
Physical Health	• What am I happy about in terms of my physical health and fitness? • How do I envision my perfect fitness/health/body? • How does my current lifestyle support/oppose this image? • I have achieved my perfect fitness/health/body, what practices and routines am I following?
External Factors	• Who are the people in my circle that *lift me up*? • What is the ideal experience I dream of having? • What are the experiences I am uncomfortable with and, therefore, avoid? • How do I need to challenge myself to grow and improve?

QUEST FOR MASTERY

The world of sports is dominated by the energy and ambition of 20-somethings. They have the speed, the power and the agility to produce top performance. They have the time to work on themselves and many have the vision to become the best in the world. Sometimes we even see some outliers who have barely finished school yet are already crushing it on World Championship and Olympic stages.

At a first glance it might look like the closer athletes are to turning 30 the higher the chance they will end their competitive careers soon. In fact, the journey that is often expected of an athlete is to put in the foundation through school and college, focus on the sports career during 20s and move on with "the rest of life," work and family around their 30s.

It's entertaining to talk about gold medals, world records and breaking the limits, but what is often left behind are the mental and emotional struggles that athletes face as they put their entire lives on hold in pursuit of the dream. These struggles tend to amplify when athletes make the transition from focusing on their sport careers to focusing on making a living. Many find it hard to slow down and adjust their competitive nature to fit with the rest of the non-athletic world.

How come so many athletes who have been in their prime during their 20s lose connection with that athletic past? Do people lose their personalities during this transition? Or do they lose confidence and resilience over time?

Not necessarily. Among the legion of energized, focused and dedicated 20-somethings are a few outcasts, outliers of a different kind. Athletes who have been in the game for a long time and each year are raising the bar for what it means to be at the top of the game. They are energetic and full of ambition yet remain calm and reserved. They are focused and committed to delivering top performance, but also have a rich world outside the arena of sports. While it might seem as though they have found a secret ingredient or a youth elixir, there is a better explanation—they all have achieved mastery in resilience.

Who are these outliers? And how does resilience develop over time? Does being resilient mean the same in your 20s as it does in your 50s?

RESILIENT ATHLETE'S LIFE PATH

For an athlete, the ability to weather the storms of everyday life often comes through sport. When everything around is stressful and turbulent, fitness is usually that one area that is reliable and provides stable ground. Active lifestyle, consistent training schedule, physical condition, health, body awareness, all of this can give the strength that athletes need to navigate tough and vulnerable times. Moreover, physical well-being can act as a stepping-stone to achieve balance across all four resilience domains. The domains, stay healthy throughout life, develop self-awareness and learn to better regulate emotions. Gather experience to accept external factors, and, of course, stay confident in the face of adversity.

What separates resilient athletes from the rest is that regardless of when they jumped on the train (in school or shortly before retiring), they continue to maintain that athletic lifestyle in joyful times and through hard patches. For some, this lifestyle means racing (competitive or not), whereas for others daily exercise is a hobby. **The most important thing is that these athletes managed to integrate sport into their lives, instead of sacrificing it for the sake of other life priorities.**

Often, this path starts in early childhood with the idea of an active lifestyle being practiced within the family. A lot of children will try several different sports (also at the same time) before the first few years of school to find something that sparks their interest, and helps to control the overflow of physical energy, of course. At this point, training is usually geared towards community, free play, and developing general athleticism (coordination, balance, agility).

Around the age of 10 to 15 kids who have been active across multiple sports will begin to outshine those who have specialized in one particular sport. That result is to a big extent thanks to functional strength and body coordination that they developed as a result of practicing different movements. In early teens, coaches pay close attention to dynamic exercises as part of a warm-up for every practice, as well as proper technique. These, seemingly simple exercises, serve as the key piece for long-term injury prevention.

The period of time between late-teens and mid 20s is when children turn into adults. They grow in size and strength, so training becomes more serious with a focus on mastering sport-specific abilities and skills (including team skills). On many occasions, this is when injuries start to show up due to a disorganized approach to training. However, athletes who have established a strong foundation in previous years will be able to improve more and have a much greater chance of reaching their full potential. Besides physical training, at this point in time, athletes also begin to develop their character, their personal standards and values, self-control and emotional regulation through participation in various competitions, and resistance to external factors by navigating the uncertainty associated with competing against others.

Things get blurry once athletes leave school/college and begin their independent lives. Many drop out and let their physical well-being go as a result of newfound responsibilities and lack of time. However, those who succeed in creating a lifestyle around sport go on to continue active training—for performance or pleasure. Of course, it is not easy to combine training with work, family and other commitments, but athletes who persevere typically have developed a profound love for fitness and movement and, therefore, go to great lengths to keep those practices in their lives. That includes establishing good habits that contribute to long-term health and surrounding yourself with like-minded individuals to support and motivate each other.

Thanks to a big base of fitness accumulated over the years, more experienced athletes do not really need that much volume to maintain a good fitness level, unless they are professionals training for the Olympics. What they can do instead is develop the purpose behind training, a vision that spans beyond performance which will be relevant even after the physiological peak.

For any athlete such "personal reinvention" should become a continuous process and happen in the background. Not just once.

Developing a purpose is not a quick process. It should not be sketched out due to an existential crisis. Much like with creating a habit, finding purpose is about trying new things and pivoting as you go.

Up until late 30s (or early 40s), a lot of training might have been motivated by goals and achieving peak performance. However, with this form of motivation, performance will inevitably start to diminish. It might not happen right away or drastically, but enough to notice that recovery gradually becomes longer, and adaptation is not as efficient. It is very humbling to accept the fact that you probably will not be as fast as you used to be, but it is also unrealistic and unfair to compare yourself at 40, 50, or 60 to where you were in your 20s. Nor does that comparison serve any purpose. Yes, it's a difficult point in athletes' lives, but life goes on. Athletes who persist are those who have formed a strong understanding of why they exercise so that all that fitness built over several decades is used for the greater good instead of being left to decline.

Getting really good at a particular sport or discipline (like running 5,000m or a marathon) requires athletes to specialize and be good at following orders, sticking to a program, listening to the coach, and checking all the boxes. However, over a longer period of time, athletes might do all of the right things but this will not work out the way they envisioned it because success is always internal. We decide what we want from our lives, so it does not make sense to give control over what we should do to anyone else. **Becoming the best version of yourself is bigger than just breaking a personal record or winning a gold medal.** It requires athletes to be more entrepreneurial, go out into the world, experiment, and find what's best for them instead of trying to fit into artificial standards. Decline of performance is not the end, but rather a beginning. The time between late-30s and late-60s is an opportunity to gather experience and perspective. Experience setting new challenges, trying out various competition formats (i.e., adventure or team races), participating in events that require travel or even practicing different sports altogether.

Achieving high levels of performance is not to be confused with being resilient. An athlete might be in peak condition, but running on reserves due to a poor diet, lack of sleep, stressful schedule, or too much intense exercise. Regardless of the purpose behind training, health is the only thing that matters. Without good health, we can only dream of all the great things we *could* have done in life. Resilient athletes are healthy, active, full of energy, and competitive even in older age (beyond 70s), because throughout their lives they have made contributions that would enable such lifestyle. They played the long game and always considered which habits promote long-term health and what training contributes to longevity in sport, instead of looking for pleasure or short-term gains. Intentional or not, these factors are what enables athletes to lead an active and joyful life.

AGE (YEARS)	CHARACTER STRENGTHS	EMOTIONAL WELL-BEING & REGULATION	PHYSICAL HEALTH	EXTERNAL WORLD
>10	Develop basic character traits	Become aware of various emotions	Engage in different activities to develop a variety of skills	Practice building social connections
10–15	Find passion and personal strengths	Learn to control emotions and focus on a certain activity	Build foundational strength and develop endurance, agility	Find a support network (coach, teammates)
15–25	Develop work ethic, discipline, consistency	Learn to regulate emotions, practice self-awareness and relaxation	Build specific strength, speed, and endurance gradually to prevent burnout	Practice dealing with uncertainty, find a mentor
25–40	Find purpose, establish personal standards and values to live by	Learn strategies to 'control' the mind and focus attention	Adopt a structured approach to training, establish good habits to build foundation of long-term health	Become a part of like-minded community
40–70	Find joy beyond performance	Develop and leverage empowering beliefs to prevent loss of motivation	Maintain consistent endurance and strength exercise regimen to extend the duration of active years	Search for new experiences to expand your perspective, be a mentor to someone
70+	Sharpen the growth mindset	Practice self-awareness and regulation	Stay active, engage in consistent strength training to maintain the quality of life, and prevent muscle loss	Become a part of community to support younger generation

Resilience lifecycle. Development goals for each of the four domains over the course of a lifetime.

MIDLIFE CRISIS IN YOUR 30S?

Our focus, goals and ambitions change as life unfolds. An age milestone, a job promotion, starting a family or even something as tangible as buying a car (or a house), these life checkpoints act as triggers to evaluate where we are and how far we have come. Sometimes, such evaluation takes an unexpected turn. *I have achieved my aspirations, so what's next? I am not where I expected to be, this isn't working. I have tried it all, but nothing works.*

The idea of a midlife crisis originated back in the 1960s when psychologists started to notice and study the changes in thinking patterns associated with ageing. These changes included feelings of remorse, sadness about lack of accomplishments in life, or emptiness after achieving big milestones. Often, these feelings lead to a desire to make drastic changes in life. While such self-confidence and existential concerns were mostly noticed in individuals aged 45 to 65, nowadays nobody is immune to it.

Sport is the arena where such existential crises are more prone to flourish. Merging the high-speed world of physical performance with the pedestrian world of everyone else is never easy regardless of whether you are in your 30s or your 60s. There are a myriad of reasons why people become less active with age and even more reasons why they do not pick up sports later in life. Professional athletes struggle to find the motivation to continue to exercise after ending their careers. Competitive amateurs find it hard to carve out time from work and family to train for a big race. Self-coached enthusiasts burn out after pushing a little too hard too soon. People who never exercised struggle to begin because they are "not made for sports."

> *Being a resilient athlete doesn't mean you haven't missed a single workout in your life. Nor does it mean that you have to do some form of sport in school to become one.*

Leading an active, fulfilling lifestyle is a continuous process in which the only thing that matters is the present moment. How far have you progressed? Which age group in the resilience lifecycle does your lifestyle suit? Are you happy with it? What will you decide to do about it?

In essence, a midlife crisis is the quest for that present moment, a hidden desire to become the best version of yourself. When faced with existential concerns and looking for an outlet, people frequently rediscover exercise, often appreciating fitness more than those active since childhood. From their new perspective, they realize something: it is not running away from problems that provides us with that rejuvenating feeling of rebirth, but running towards something better—growth and progress.

THE BEST TIME TO START IS NOW: RICH ROLL'S BATTLE AGAINST MIDDLE AGE

At the age of forty, Rich Roll was far from his prime. A promising swimmer in college, he felt lost in the world of corporate law, struggled with substance abuse and generally was in horrible physical shape. The extra fifty pounds that accumulated throughout the years was a daily reminder of the trajectory his life was on. But that was about to change.

On the eve of his 40th birthday, Rich found himself struggling to climb a single flight of stairs—panting and in pain. With his lifestyle fueled by fast-food and alcohol, a heart attack was certainly in the cards…and that was *with* his competitive background. That health scare (or "epiphany" as Rich calls it) was a trigger that set in motion an internal growth mechanism and paved the way not only to recovery, but also resilience. In the years that followed Rich has gradually climbed his way back, became an accomplished vegan ultra-endurance athlete and rediscovered his passion for health, vitality, and fitness in the process. In his 50s, he feels much stronger than he was in his 20s and, more importantly, he feels a bigger purpose behind all of that fitness.

It was not a quick fix, nor was it a smooth ride. It took Rich a few years to rebuild his fitness and develop the stamina to be able to even begin taking part in endurance events. It took several more years to overcome additional setbacks that were happening in his life, one of which being the financial pressure from leaving a corporate job. However, all of that adversity gave him the opportunity for growth and helped him develop resilience across all four domains—not just physically. By the time Rich had accomplished some of his biggest endurance feats, he was able to connect the dots and realize that fitness was never the goal. Instead, it was part of who he was. A rock that he could rely on throughout life and a stable ground that he had lost touch with after college. So, the journey of rebuilding fitness was really the journey of self-discovery for him.

Rich was able to pivot and find the answer to the middle age dilemma. He is a great example that you can overcome anything at any age, as long as you begin and commit.

Resilience has several domains and people might approach mastering it from different angles. A resilient athlete is not born or made during his or her teenage years. Starting to exercise later in life does not mean these new-born athletes have missed the train. It only means they are in a "younger" age group of resilience lifecycle and should go through more phases before reaching mastery.

For example, a 50-year-old beginner runner with minimum experience who wants to finish a marathon has some training and adjusting to do before the body becomes strong enough to cover the distance. On the resilient athlete timeline, these people are in their early teens and, thus, should focus on building foundational strength and mobility before trying to run hundreds of miles in preparation for a marathon. This does not mean, however, that it will take them years to get to the late-teens phase and start adding volume. Thanks to decades of walking and day-to-day activities this process will happen faster. Often what is required are a few weeks (or months) of easy exercise, base strength, and mobility exercises to create a base that will support a large training volume ahead.

Even though people who engage in sports later in life have some catching up to do in terms of physical well-being, they might be quite mature in other resilience domains. Thanks to life experience, these people often are more conscious of their emotional well-being, have a purpose behind embarking on a fitness journey, and maybe even built resistance to external factors (like opinions or pressure). Which is why we cannot look at things in black and white, be it lifestyle, fitness, mindset, or even personality. Any experience we have in life requires all sides of us to be balanced in maturity.

The path to achieving that balance and mastering resilience is long and treacherous. It is peppered with distractions and opportunities to do what's easy, to have an emotional outbreak instead of learning to self-regulate, or have a cheat meal instead of making oneself a smoothie. As satisfying as it is in the moment, settling for those appealing disturbances, either emotionally or physically, takes the attention away from what is missing and tips life off balance.

BEGINNER'S MIND AND THE FOUR STAGES OF MASTERY

Experience in sports can be both a blessing and a curse. While it does create a foundation for an active lifestyle, chasing after a goal can also lead athletes to make choices against long-term health, like training through pain or illness, or adopting an intense training schedule on top of stressful day-to-day life. Moreover, doing something new and different tends to be harder for more experienced people because they are often used to their routines and more hesitant to change. For example, an athlete who is used to doing a lot of high intensity training might be more reluctant to adopt a more balanced, yet sustainable training program, due to concerns over losing the progress made so far.

People with minimum experience, on the other hand, whether in their teens or their 50s, typically do not have a problem experimenting with new training methodologies or routines. They have a more relaxed worldview and approach things from a beginner's perspective, happy about little achievements, get motivated by progress instead of immediate results, and recognize that there is a long way ahead which does not grow shorter by standing still.

Everyone starts somewhere and any learning journey passes through a phase where an individual is not doing things right. To go through that phase and eventually get better, we need to get comfortable being very uncomfortable. To make mistakes and see them as opportunities to get better, and to be willing to accept and appreciate the unpleasant and not give up. When we remove the comparison with other people or even ourselves, that is when we start to learn and become more empowered to make a change.

Zen Buddhism calls this idea *shoshin*—the beginner's mind. It emphasizes the value of humility and curiosity when learning a certain subject, even if you are already well-educated in it. Looking at things from the point of view of a beginner helps you to stay open to making mistakes, finding and analyzing patterns, and, therefore, grow. This concept is relevant for learning a subject, practicing a skill, and almost everything else in life. In fact, athletes make mistakes all the time—that is just the nature of progress. Maybe the training program was too ambitious, there was unexpected cold or muscle pain, the taper did not work out as planned or the race did not go as expected. All of that is precious experience and counts towards becoming more resilient in the future.

Let's imagine for a moment that resilience itself is a skill which we can learn and master. Emotional regulation, resistance to external stimuli, adopting healthy lifestyle habits or even staying true to purpose and navigating a midlife crisis are not as easy as learning to whistle or do the moonwalk. I agree, but with enough practice these skills can become second nature as well. How would you go about doing it? And where would you start?

In practice, there are four stages of learning a new skill[1] that we pass through on our way to mastery. This process requires that individuals are initially unaware of the skill and their lack of proficiency in it, unconscious of their incompetence. As they recognize that gap (become conscious of the incompetence), they put conscious effort to learn the skill and apply it (conscious competence). Eventually, after enough practice, the skill becomes second nature and an individual is able to perform it without thinking about how to do it right. That is when he or she has acquired unconscious competence.

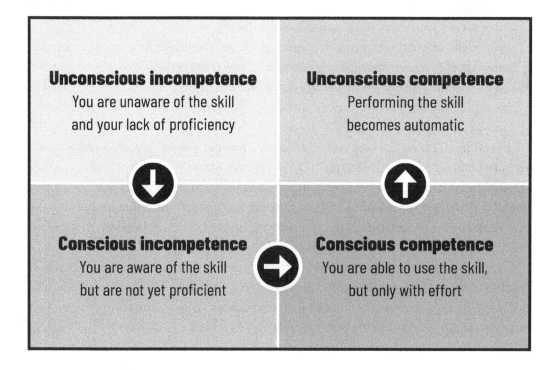

Four stages of competence model.

---

1   In reference to the Stages of Competence Model introduced by Noel Burch in the 1970s

Let's use a hypothetical triathlete as an example to visualize this process of skill learning. Say hello to Mark, a 37-year-old hobby-triathlete who swims twice a week in preparation for his first half Ironman triathlon. He can already cover the race distance of 1.2 miles (1.9K) but is struggling to get faster at it. Like many others, Mark used to swim during his childhood to be water-safe, but never took up competitive swimming as a profession until now.

Swimming is a good example to illustrate the process of learning, because it is a very technique-driven sport. A lot of the process for becoming a better swimmer relies on reducing drag that the body produces in the water and making smooth and coordinated strokes. More often than not, an unfit experienced swimmer will still be faster in the water than a very fit non-swimmer because experienced swimmers practice the mechanics of the stroke over many years and for them smoothness is second nature. Sure, there are some details that even elite swimmers consciously focus on improving in their practice, but those are minute in comparison with the overall skill level.

Learning any skill starts with self-awareness. Or, for beginners, the lack of it. Mark, who has been swimming on and off for some time, might consider himself a decent swimmer. He is able to stay above the water, make strokes, remember to breathe, and not drown. However, he is not aware of small technical aspects of the freestyle technique and mistakes he is making that slow him down. In other words, he is unconscious of his incompetence. In fact, many swimmers and triathletes in his position try to add more intensity to improve fitness hoping to become faster and more enduring in the water. This helps a little, but besides adding a lot of fatigue such improvements are temporary and the moment athletes take a break, such "swim fitness" takes a nosedive.

Mark, who doesn't have much time to swim every week, asked a coach for advice. He requested that Mark film himself underwater, and as expected, there were a few major flaws in Mark's stroke technique that worked against him. In particular, he looked too far ahead as he swam, which shifted the balance more to the back and caused his legs to sink. On top of that, he also crossed the midline of the body with his front arm causing the legs to compensate and swing in a different direction. After reviewing the footage with the coach and receiving feedback, Mark became aware of his mistakes and the deficit he needed to address to improve his speed and endurance. He thus moved into a conscious incompetence phase.

Next came the phase of active learning. To address some inefficiencies, the coach advised a few drills (simple isolated exercises) that focus on improving body positioning in the water and correct hand entry. The purpose behind these drills was to mimic the correct movement pattern and consciously repeat it multiple times until it became automatic. It did require a lot of focused effort for Mark because the correct movement felt unnatural to him. However, that was just a phase in learning the correct mechanics, and with conscious practice, he became more comfortable with it.

Eventually, this process of actively thinking about how a particular movement feels during the drill helped Mark to create a mind muscle connection and gradually replicate that movement in his actual swimming. With consistent practice, he has improved that skill of body positioning and hand entry to the point when he no longer needs concentration to get it right. Mark noticed that he was able to maintain steady effort for longer without adding more intensity into his schedule, which is what he was after in preparation for the half Ironman triathlon.

Those few drills have by no means created a perfect technique, but what's important is that Mark's form did improve. As he continues to actively look for mistakes and become conscious of how things should feel, his results will continue to improve. For the same purpose, technique drills are used across many sports to instill correct movement patterns and recruit muscles in a more efficient way. Quite often improper form and biomechanics is what puts a limit on how fit an athlete can get and how much of that fitness translates to athletic performance.

We can apply the same style of thinking to building resilience. It is not something that a lucky few are born with, but is a skill that everyone can learn, practice and master. Everyone can take matters into their own hands, evaluate what's missing, become more self-aware and take conscious steps towards improvement. Continually rediscover and improve yourself, bounce back, try new things, and develop one small area at a time.

The key to learning any skill is to adopt a beginner's mindset to overcome the paralyzing belief of "I'm not made for this."

Accept the fact that you will be at level 0 when you start something. Without going through the first levels, you will not get to the next ones. You start as a beginner, so treat yourself like one. Remember to focus on the progress, so that this beginnerism does not hold you back.

In the previous chapter, you discovered what it takes to be a resilient athlete. You might have also taken note of your strong sides as well as gaps that prevent you from becoming the best version of yourself. Whatever those areas are, consider them skills that you can learn, practice, and eventually, master.

The exercise at the end of this chapter will guide you through the phases of skill mastery and set you on the path to develop resilience across all four domains, from personal attributes to emotional regulation to physical fitness to being strong against external factors. It will help you to evaluate your level of resilience, determine what is missing and begin taking conscious actions to close the gap between where you are and where you want to be and become a more grounded, confident, and well-rounded athlete as a result.

EXERCISE: SHOW ME THE PATH

Starting in early childhood and staying active through life is an ideal scenario, but this does not mean that if you are late to the party you cannot hop on the moving train and become a resilient athlete. It is never too late to start—the earlier you do, the more time you will spend investing in yourself.

You might be starting your athletic journey when you are in your 40s or resuming after a few decades of no activity. If that is the case, don't worry. Feeling like you do not belong is normal and signals that you are stepping into the unknown. It is only by embracing what's uncomfortable that we are able to make a meaningful shift in our lives. Everyone started somewhere and the best time to start something is always now. After all, it is not like you are starting from scratch. You might already be resilient in your ability to self-regulate and have a strong character, but your physical well-being is a little out of balance. It could also be vice versa, you are really fit, but have a hard time figuring out what to do next.

The exercise ahead helps us to map out the journey to becoming a resilient athlete. Think of it as building a skill and use the process to determine your competence level in each of the resilience domains and the steps you need to take to master them. Most importantly, be honest with yourself and maintain the beginner's mindset. Focus on one step at a time, self-awareness, resolve and building a habit. Give it time and be patient.

You have already taken a hard look at each of the resilience domains in the last chapter. Which of the four was the one you feel lags behind? Start the exercise with *that one domain* in mind and once you finish, repeat for all remaining domains.

Step 1: Self-Awareness

Just like mastering a skill, start by becoming aware of the level of "competence" you currently possess in a resilience domain. To help you assess your level, revisit the resilient athlete lifecycle shared earlier in this chapter. Be honest and answer the question which age group would I place myself in? Is it age 10–15 and I am lacking strength in my joints to support hard training? Or rather in age 15 to 25 and my endurance is subpar? Maybe I have a good foundation of strength, but struggle with maintaining a healthy lifestyle? Once you know where you are, you can see what else you need to develop in order to move ahead.

The beginning is generally the most challenging part, because often we are not aware of the fact that there are areas that need improvement or things we need to learn.

Besides asking for feedback, the best way to become self-aware is to get yourself to reflect on how things are going. Start a journaling practice—take 10 minutes every day to ask yourself challenging questions and write down your thoughts. Be open to the fact that you might have weaknesses or areas you are not handling well. Such ownership of responsibility empowers you to take action and make changes for the better. The goal of this step is to move from unconscious incompetence to conscious incompetence (understand what's missing), so focus on finding specific things that are not working and what you can do to fix them.

Here are some of the questions you might ask yourself:

1. Am I waking up in the morning ready to take on the day?
   a. What is not working for me at the moment?

2. When my mind is not in the present moment, where is it instead?
   a. What concerns me the most at the moment?
   b. What worries me most about the future?

3. What are the top three mistakes that are preventing me from showing up at my best?
   a. What influence do these mistakes have on me?
   b. How can I prevent these mistakes?
   c. What first step I can take to prevent/fix these mistakes?

4. Where do I avoid the unpleasant in order to feel comfortable?

    a.   What am I not doing that I should be doing?

    b.   What is the first decision I have to make that I have not yet made?

5. What is the one bad habit that is limiting my ability to succeed?

    a.   What am I willing to do about it?

6. What unhelpful thought patterns are limiting my personal growth?

    a.   Are these thought patterns true?

    b.   Would I teach these thought patterns to my children?

    c.   What is the true price that I am paying for engaging in these thought patterns?

    d.   What am I trying to gain by holding on to these thought patterns?

7. If I could change one thing right now, what would it be?

    a.   What is the first and easiest step I can take to kick-start this change?

Based on this self-reflection, answer these for yourself:

- What is preventing me from being a resilient athlete?
- What prevents me from being my absolute best?

STRATEGY: THE FIVE WHY APPROACH TO PERSONAL GROWTH

When dealing with pain, experiencing negative emotions, or even facing difficulties, the first gut response is often to "use a bandage" to cover up the effect and get back in shape as quickly as possible. Experiencing a headache? Pop a pill and get back to work. It is a quick way to remove a symptom but does little to prevent the disturbance from reappearing. To fully address a problem or issue, we need to identify and resolve its root cause. If we do not, it will continue to surface and will likely become worse. Kind of like fixing the leaking roof by changing the bucket, eventually the leakage will cause the roof to collapse.

It is not always obvious what the underlying issue is, which is why sometimes it takes time to fully resolve a problem. Fortunately, the Five Why process is an effective way to determine the root cause and understand how to fix it. Originally developed by Toyota in the 1970s and still used to this day, it is a great strategy to help understand what is really preventing you from moving forward in your training, business, or life as a whole. The process is as simple as it sounds:

Identify the problem. Start by defining what exactly is not right (i.e., undesired result or state). Write it down in a journal and leave plenty of space for answers. For example, *"I'm spending too much time on my phone and it's affecting my productivity and emotional state."*

Ask the first Why? Ask yourself why this problem is occurring. For example, *"Why am I spending so much time on my phone? Possible answer: Because I am using it to avoid doing the tasks that I need to."* It sounds simple, but answering it honestly requires some serious thinking. Look for answers that are backed by facts, things that have actually taken place, instead of assumptions about what could have happened. This helps you to keep the process real and avoid chasing down hypothetical problems. Also, it is important to keep emotions aside and instead take an unbiased 3rd party look at the situation.

Ask Why four more times. For each of the answers, ask further Whys in succession and frame the question in response to the answer you have just recorded. Example: *Why am I avoiding doing the tasks that I need to? Possible answer: Because I'm not in the right headspace to prepare for and overcome each task in a mindful and joyous way.* You will know that you have reached the root cause of the problem when asking Why produces no more useful responses, and you cannot go any further. An appropriate solution or habit change will then become evident.

Step 2: Resolve

Resilient people focus their energy on the things within their control, rather than fixating on factors they cannot impact. Which is why they feel empowered to make a change after seeing how their shortcomings hamper progress. This desire to change is a signal that a person is ready to enter the next stage—conscious competence.

In order to carry this momentum through, you need to act. Make the decision to resolve what is not working for you and commit to taking conscious steps to follow through. Extraordinary results do not happen from wishing or thinking or planning. If you go into something half-hearted and think *what if...*the result will not be what you expect it to be.

Here are some of the questions you can ask yourself to help discover what you can do to start moving towards where you want to be or who you want to become:

1. What has to change for me to start growing?
   a. What can I do to become 1% better every day?
   b. What one step can I take right now to improve the quality of my life?
   c. What can help me to create momentum?

2. What does the best-case scenario look like for me?
   a. How would it look like if it was easy?
   b. What one step I can take now to start making that scenario a reality?

3. What are the three accomplishments I am most proud of?
   a. What helped me achieve these accomplishments?
   b. How can I replicate and leverage that in other areas?

4. What does being the best version of myself mean to me?
5. What kind of a person will I need to become to achieve that?
   a. What beliefs do I have to develop to become that?
   b. What routines do I need to implement to become that?
   c. What skills do I need to learn to become that?

    d. Who can support me in becoming that?

    e. What resources do I have already (books, training programs, peer-groups)?

Write down one action, that if you committed to today would change your life for the better:

- What one action can I take right now to start being my absolute best?
- What one action can I take right now to start being a resilient athlete?

Extraordinary results come from taking action. Think of a decision you have already made sometime in the past, one that you hesitated to make multiple times, but you eventually did and it changed your whole life for the better. What finally got you to decide? How can you bring that same level of focus to building resilience?

To help you cultivate that desire to change, go out of your comfort zone and follow through. Answer the following four questions, keeping that one action in mind:

1. What will happen if I do commit to this one action?
2. What will not happen if I do commit to this one action?
3. What will happen if I don't commit to this one action?
4. What will not happen if I don't commit to this one action?

Step 3: Build a Habit

Once you commit to a certain action, it is time to start introducing healthy practices in each of the resilience domains and actively sticking to them until the resilient behavior becomes second nature (unconscious competence phase). Do it gradually and add good habits and practices one by one to avoid becoming overwhelmed by change.

In this last step, put yourself in a position where you are forced to practice. Introduce routines, find accountability partners, set reminders, use a journal, whatever you need to do to make sure you stick with the process. **The practice of learning will never end, so it is important to have a process to constantly refine your skill.**

Athletes can put tons of time into practicing technique, but if they do not analyze their mistakes, they will not improve much. Same with resilience. The key to creating a lifestyle that is sustainable is what they call "deliberate practice." Instead of mindlessly repeating the same actions over and over, we need to be more focused and analytical about them, review what went well, what didn't and how to improve. Ideally, with a mentor, a coach, or an accountability partner.

Write down what you can do to incorporate deliberate practice into your daily life:

- What am I already really good at that comes naturally to me?
- What makes that skill second nature and how can I replicate it in other areas?
- How can I make sure I am at my absolute best every day?
- What systems can I put in place to automate the right behavior?
- How will I know if I am making progress?
- How can I keep myself accountable?

You will find specific strategies, tips, and self-improvement actions that you can implement in the upcoming chapters. The rest of Part I is devoted to character strengths, emotional well-being, and the external world, whereas Parts II and III cover the area of physical well-being.

THE SUPERCOMPENSATION EFFECT

"Train hard, fight easy." An age-old adage that has found its way from the ranks of Suvorov's army to well beyond the battlefield in the everyday lives of elite performers.

What is one thing great athletes, actors, and businesspeople have in common that lets them produce truly outstanding performances even under immense pressure? Going to the far sides of the comfort zone. Much like soldiers in the army, top performers practice at higher intensity and in more challenging conditions than what they'll face when they compete or perform. All with the purpose of making the pressure of the big day feel easier and more manageable.

The process of growing stronger and more resilient in response to stress is in our nature. In fact, in sports science it is called **supercompensation** and is an effect where the body builds itself up stronger in anticipation of facing more adversity ahead. The same effect takes place in our minds as we go through thousands of stressful situations during our lifetime and adapt by learning how to cope with them. So, it is quite likely that we are able to handle a problem or a challenge much better the second or third time we are facing it, compared to our initial response.

What is harder, however, is to navigate a new situation. Doing something we have not done before is uncomfortable even if we are proficient in the skill. Besides the intense thought process taking place in our brain (analyze the situation, assess risks, make a decision), there is always an element of uncertainty. There is no guarantee for a specific result and potential for more challenges. It is like going on a 3-hour-long bike ride along the route you have prepared on your phone and halfway through the session the phone crashes leaving you with no directions. While you are proficient in riding a bike, you are not sure how to get home and need to navigate by signs or ask for directions. This will involve some stopping or even turning around after riding in the wrong direction, so the session might end up more stressful and less qualitative than expected.

It is no wonder that stepping out of your comfort zone feels intimidating. It is difficult for someone who has the opportunity to take it easy and do what is certain instead. *Who wants to go running when it's raining outside? I only have 30 minutes, I better train when I have more time. What's the purpose of training if all races are being cancelled anyway?* Whenever we don't push against the resistance of doubt, low self-esteem, and confidence, we stop growing. In fact, we slide down instead, because life doesn't remain still. It is inevitable that we will face more challenges in life and if we remain at the current level of resilience, it will get increasingly harder to handle situations in the future. Often this is the reason why people become trapped in the past and use their mistakes, rejections, and disappointments as a measure of what they can achieve in the future, thus not living fully and not taking advantage of opportunities.

Here's the catch. **Any given moment of our life—be it an athletic challenge or a life event—requires all stages of us to come together.** All of the experiences we had and everything we learned when we were 20, 40 or even 60 years old do count because they got us to that particular moment. So, every time we avoid doing something because it's challenging, we rob ourselves of the opportunity to become stronger and handle adversity that lies ahead better. Our life is one big preparation journey for the next event, performance, or a peak. We make progress towards those, one small supercompensation at a time. Of course, as the time passes, limits become less physical. However, we should not stop breaking them.

The purpose behind taking on any new experience is the same reason why we push ourselves in training. Self-efforts that we make stretch our physical and mental capacity and drive the body and mind to adapt. Top performers thrive on challenges because they make them stronger, more resilient, and able to handle the storms of life better. It sets them up for success, generates energy and creates the spark to impact and lead others.

PROFOUND EXPERIENCE

Not any experience has the power to create an optimal, exciting, and fulfilling life. It needs to be profound and challenging to make a meaningful shift.

We may find it anywhere, at the finish line of a marathon, on a wedding day, after a particularly stressful day at work, or even when someone makes an innocent joke about us. Butterflies in the stomach. Feelings of euphoria, timelessness or determination. Even excitement about breaking through something whether that be your limitations, concerns, stereotypes, or adversity. A weird mix of emotions that is hard to describe, let alone control.

It is an intense sense of accomplishment and a strong gust of change that comes with energy, focus and readiness to conquer the world. We seek this sensational state, but at the same time are also intimidated by it. That signal that something has shifted in life, as if things will never be the same, is usually followed by a sense of empowerment or positive affirmations, such as: *I can do hard things, I will do whatever it takes, I won't take it anymore, I will prove them wrong.*

Abraham Maslow called this feeling the Peak Experience—an occasion when the state of mind becomes considerably different to a normal state in response to a certain life event.[1] These are not everyday events and are often described as exhilarating moments of pure joy and fulfillment. Moments when the rest of the world fades away. Moments that we tend to carry in our memories for a long time and even reflect on as turning points in our lives.

Peak Experiences are exciting, exhilarating and elevating. They might manifest in the form of events, interactions or activities that lead to a personal realization, feeling of success or a sense of reaching one's full potential.

Some of the most powerful factors that forge a Peak Experience are:

- **Complete presence:** A sense of unity with oneself and the environment. Often Peak Experiences are called spiritual, because individuals feel connected with their purpose and even lose track of time.

- **Energy:** A feeling like you have reached the top of the world, jubilation, accomplishment, peak strength or even adrenalin rush.

---

1   American psychologist Abraham Maslow introduced the concept of Peak Experiences in his 1943 paper "A Theory of Human Motivation" and in his 1964 book "Religions, Values, and Peak Experiences".

- **Timing:** The effect experience has on us is magnified by the time it takes to unfold. Finishing a marathon is not only about crossing the finish line after a 3, 4 or 5 hours of running. It is the culmination of months of physical and mental training.

- **Uniqueness:** Rarity of the experience leads to an increased awareness of its value. We tend to remember and cherish individual moments more, because statistically they might never happen again.

A profound experience requires focus, time, and preparation, and the unfolding of it is not always positive or smooth. It takes courage to face adversity and self-discipline to stay on course, but when hard work manifests into a breakthrough or an empowering realization (i.e., believing in yourself), it's like rocket fuel for our growth and resilience. The more effort we put forth in the lead-up to an event, the more profound the experience will be because we are more emotionally attached. That, in turn, helps us to connect better with our authentic self.

Sounds like a great thing to do with your life, but how do you craft experiences that make you grow instead of tearing you down in the process? By cultivating aspects that create a profound experience through daily rituals and mindset shifts.

CIRCLE OF LIFE

Whatever we consistently tell ourselves becomes the story that, over the course of many repetitions, we start to believe in. Someone who does not feel confident or worthy of success will look for every opportunity to complain, feel weak, or give up.

The difference between success and failure comes down to how much effort we put in, not by whether we are lucky or not. People who expect to fail will hinder themselves in what they can achieve right from the start. Doubts limit our beliefs, which limits our actions and, as a result, the outcomes we get. Eventually, such people will find evidence to confirm the doubts by making a mistake or failing, consciously or not. Even a single doubt that runs through the mind of an athlete before the race can be the deciding factor for them not giving his or her best.

Both our potential in life and the outcomes we get are not determined by the outside world. They are not dictated by our economic situation, not by the opinions shared by influencers, and not even by our past. The results we get are only dependent on the strength of our characters and the actions we take. Very often, people achieve great things because they didn't know those things would be difficult or impossible.

"They did not know it was impossible, so they did it."

— MARK TWAIN

When people tell themselves, *"I can't do it, it's not me, I'm not cut for this,"* they are saying it based on the setbacks they have had in the past. They might have tried to do something similar before but fallen short of expectations. And the more times they were unsuccessful, the stronger this negative belief became.

However, falling short of expectations does not equal the inability to do that thing. Athletes do that all the time. They shoot for the Moon, miss it and sometimes hit a star. Ambition is part of what drives the process of discovery and self-actualization. What distinguishes resilient athletes is their perseverance. They continue to try, because they are aware that what happens to us, and the results that we get in life, are both pieces of a jigsaw puzzle. Once the rest of the puzzle is solved, the missing piece fits without a hitch.

The intensity and the impact a particular experience has on us is not a factor of luck. Instead, we ourselves hold the power to design it. Those life-changing realizations and breakthroughs we have as a result of life events or interactions are manifestations of a longer setup process that I like to call the *Circle of Life*.

The strength of our character determines our beliefs and ambitions. Our ability to focus on those (emotional fitness) affects our mental state (flow), which influences the actions we take and the effort we put in. The magnitude of our action impacts the outcome (experience), which, in turn, shapes our beliefs and ambitions further. The circle starts again.

The key factor that enables this transformative process is our physical well-being. When we are healthy, strong, energized, and connected with our bodies, there is no limit to what we can achieve. We're more confident, able to control emotions better, and can better remain focused on important tasks and activities. As a result, have more meaningful and transformative experiences.

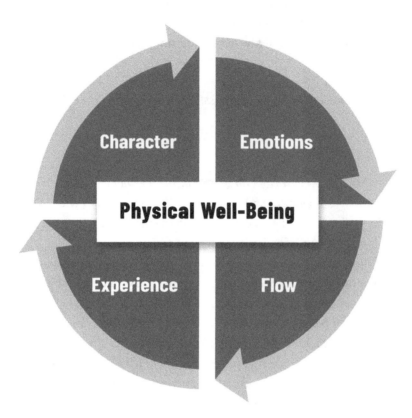

The Circle of Life.

This setup process originates in our mind. We form certain beliefs about our potential and ambitions based on how we see and interact with the world. These beliefs are driven by our character attributes: purpose, vision, goals, theme for life, strengths, weaknesses, personal values, and standards.

As we interact with the external world, we are exposed to different situations and opinions that make us feel a certain way. Maybe it is a stressful situation that causes feelings of anxiety or angst. Or we hear someone's opinion that we disagree with and it triggers frustration and fury. This baggage we carry in response to an event or interaction is nothing more than negative emotions that prevent us from looking at the bright side and feeling motivated rather than discouraged. Even though we cannot always control which thoughts pop into our heads, we do get to choose what we focus on. That comes from our ability to self-regulate.

With enough self-reflection practice we can start to recognize feelings and emotions triggered in response to external occurrences, interactions or even our own thought process. Once we develop that competence, we can take the appropriate action based on our gained intelligence. In particular, evaluate the situation in relation to personal goals and ambitions (recognize destructive emotions and behaviors, notice provocation attempts, etc.) and consider what the most productive course of action will be.

This capacity to quiet down the chatter of the external world and focus on what's important is called emotional fitness. Instead of paralyzing us like fear or doubt does, it creates more time and headspace to be fully present and translate our beliefs, ambitions, and goals into action. Adapting to circumstances in such a way not only breaks the cycle of reacting to life, but also breeds the courage and confidence needed to get out of your comfort zone and bring your A game.

In fact, immersing yourself fully in the experience is one of the key factors to achieve the flow,[1] a state of absolute certainty about your abilities. When athletes are in the flow, they are completely engaged with their body and are able to concentrate without distraction, produce their best performance, and more importantly, feel indestructible. Nothing feels impossible when you are in the flow state of mind.

What kind of outcome would you expect from someone who brings his or her best self to the experience—be it a race, a day at work or even a date with someone special? Exactly, that person will put a substantial effort in, go the extra mile and deliver his or her best performance against all odds. And this outcome will only raise their self-confidence and motivation to achieve even more.

Our character attributes, emotional fitness and ability to enter the flow state define the quality of life events and interactions we get to have and by virtue of those, define our life. As we interpret those experiences, we unconsciously assign labels and meanings to them (i.e., pain, pleasure, joy, sadness), which either confirms or weakens beliefs about our potential and ambitions. That is where the circle starts again. Stronger belief leads to more focus, more

---

1   In reference to Mihaly Csikszentmihalyi's book "Flow: The Psychology of Optimal Experience"

action, and more profound experience, which strengthens the belief even further. Vice versa, every hero's journey ends at the starting point with the magic elixir, the knowledge, skills, or routines for how to live a better life. All with the purpose of enabling harder challenges ahead and growing even more.

CASE STUDY: "I'M GETTING TOO OLD FOR THIS"

Meet Adam, an athlete that I coached who struggled with improving his results. He has developed a belief that at 48 he is just not as fast as he used to be and running long distances becomes increasingly risky for people of his age. While he was very active in his teens and even was on the college basketball team, he let go of active sports to focus on his corporate career and family. That is until he picked up running shortly before turning 40. Four marathons and six half marathons later he thought he had reached his peak—full distance in 4 hours and 30 minutes was the barrier he could not break through.

His commitment was strong. Be it summer or winter, he was putting in the miles whatever the weather. However, his training was nothing special, just a free plan he found online that called for a run 3–4 times per week with a gradual increase in duration. The intensity was not specified, so more often than not, Adam pushed himself to put a solid workout in. Many times, he pushed it too far—to the point of persistent discomfort and pain because he was concerned whether or not he was getting maximum benefits during his busy schedule.

Lingering pain he had developed in the knee eventually led to frustration and thoughts of "becoming too old for this." That meant that his experiences (pain and less than expected marathon results) had affected his belief about what he is capable of, affected what he focused on (pain instead of progress), and affected his willingness to take action. *What if I make it worse?* Such thinking locked him in a victim mindset and signaled his brain to expect failure. He didn't put enough training in and didn't get the results he hoped for, which confirmed his belief that he must be getting too old for running.

This "go hard or go home" approach is a common theme among amateur athletes. By chasing quick results, they often skip foundational steps that help to sustain the stress of a consistent training schedule. For Adam (and many of his peers), it was a question of acceptance instead of performance. The first thing he had to do was to let go of the idea of measuring himself against some artificial standards, like a sub-4 finish or his 10K personal best in high school, and instead focus on immersing himself in the process. The only standard we set for him was whether or not what he did brought him joy.

Besides this headwork, Adam also adapted a more consistent and balanced training regimen. Instead of running hard for three days a week, he gradually switched to running six days per week for 20–40 minutes each day. It felt like a significant step-down for him and his ego, as most of those days were easy running that felt like walking, but besides running, each session included a form of mobility, strength, core, or conditioning exercises to make him more physically well-rounded.

Within a month, Adam felt the first signs of progress. His knee pain had diminished, and he realized that removing the pressure he had carried brought back the joy that made him fall in love with running eight years ago. Within half a year, he was able to gradually increase his training volume and finished a marathon in 3 hours and 42 minutes—beating his personal best by close to 50 minutes. More importantly, this was not even the focus anymore. Throughout the training process, Adam grew more excited about his progress and started to look for ways to integrate his newfound fitness with his other passion, traveling. The experience of pushing past the limitations reinvigorated his belief about what he's capable of and energized him to consider taking up other challenges.

The weight that athletes put on results and meeting certain standards often creates immense pressure. Why not alleviate that and instead of feeling frustrated about not meeting expectations, become grateful for all the things that happened that led to this point? We can still set goals to strive for, but they should be realistic. Being the best version of yourself or being a resilient athlete does not mean that you have to beat your personal best all the time. It means to have more energy to follow a cause that is meaningful and not spend that energy for some fitness benefit.

The purpose of completing a challenge (marathon, Ironman triathlon, etc.) is not to smash a personal best, but to have a profound experience. Maybe see other places and expand your perspective. Or maybe even build an empowering community and lead by showing an example of a healthy lifestyle.

What are you passionate about? What can you do with your fitness? Which sport you always wanted to try but were so focused on beating your PRs?

We can pivot our lives at any stage in the Circle to craft a bigger purpose, learn to control emotions better, practice strategies to enter the flow and even get out of our comfort zones by signing up for more unique experiences. However, what holds this circle together is physical well-being, the cornerstone of leading a better life. Those who want to thrive in life instead of just surviving, should set themselves up accordingly by optimizing their lifestyle for more energy and vitality.

In exchange, they will:

- **Character.** Stay confident and excited about executing the vision and work to accomplish goals.
- **Emotions.** Have lower stress levels, be able to better self-regulate, and keep themselves mentally aligned.
- **Flow.** Have the energy to cultivate the winner's mindset and show up at their absolute best.
- **Experience.** Have the willpower to step out of the comfort zone and try new and different things.

Fitness is about running fast or lifting heavy. It impacts the person's entire well-being: looking and feeling your best, having the energy to do what is important, having the stamina to handle physical and emotional stress, being resistant to various diseases, and having the strength and endurance to accomplish physical challenges.

However, if physical well-being is like oil for the Circle of Life, challenge is the engine that sets the entire process in motion.

THE POWER OF A CHALLENGE

Can you recall the last time you had peak experience? That moment when you got goosebumps from the excitement of doing something new? And when you were completely present and felt like you were on top of the world? I'm sure you can remember how intense it was. We're going to need that memory in Chapter 6 to dig deeper into the power of mental state, but for now it's more important to recognize what led to that experience—courage.

The thing is, as humans we strive for comfort—thanks in large to the legacy of our ancient fears of being eaten by bigger and stronger predators. Ever since hunter-gatherer times, our brain has developed an instinct to look for a safe haven. A tree branch above the ground, a cave in the middle of the Savannah or, you know, that warm cozy place inside us called the comfort zone. Many people find it hard to take big or bold enough action and, as a result, they do not generate unique and profound experiences that help to make meaningful shifts in their lives. That creates a feeling of being "stuck" in life, repeating the same pattern in the pursuit of optimization, saving time, or meeting certain standards. Never venturing into the unknown and not living up to the true potential.

The secret to becoming the best version of yourself lies in the supercompensation effect. In the same way, our body recovers quicker from a short and easy training session, a small habit, mindset, or lifestyle change is easy to handle. We do not need much energy to execute a small shift and can consistently repeat the good behavior, Just like going for an easy training session every day, many of those healthy practices put together over a prolonged period of time result in a significant lifestyle shift (think big fitness gain following a training block). So, while we might think we need a major action to make a meaningful shift in life, in reality all we need are many small consistent wins.

Since it is not in our nature to go beyond the comfort zone, we need a trigger, a moment of courage to commit to something. This is where, as a coach, I usually ask the question "When have you last challenged yourself beyond your competence? What would be a good test for you?" Stepping out of the comfort zone sets in motion the entire Circle of Life. It is uncomfortable and intimidating, so when we commit to one action, it serves as a date on the calendar towards the thing we are striving for. A good challenge complements and revives the purpose. It drives an individual to show up every day, gain momentum, and have a long-term focus in mind. It helps to quiet down the irrelevant noise and access the flow state. And then there's the excitement of the experience itself.

Be it a physical challenge—like finishing an Ironman—or a personal project, forcing yourself to consistently do things that are more uncomfortable than you are used to is a great way to put yourself in a position to create more profound experiences that will make a difference in your life. In fact, completing a challenge might also serve as a stepping stone on a longer journey of self-discovery asking, *"If I can do this, what else can I do?"* Make sure you step outside of your comfort zone even just a little bit, but more frequently. In the long term, these small steps accumulate and expand the boundaries of what is comfortable, build resilience, and bring high performance to a totally new level.

EXERCISE: THE BUCKET LIST

This exercise is about taking that first step and getting used to the idea of willingly stepping into the unknown to generate energy and kick-start the process of personal transformation. Kind of like creating the first supercompensation in the longer process of self-discovery and growth.

You might have heard the term "bucket list" already. It's a list of things you wish to achieve, dreams you want to fulfill, and life experiences you want to have whether that might be big or small, purposeful or random. Having such a list helps to remind you of what matters in your life so that you can spend time acting on it instead of being distracted by minute stressors of everyday life.

Life shouldn't be all serious all the time. Having a dream or a crazy adventure in mind adds a bit of thrill to your life and might even help you to discover new passions. Even though many people set goals for themselves, creating a bucket list is different. It's like planning all the highlights of your life and is an incredibly insightful exercise. Often, setting audacious goals and planning epic adventures makes people more enthusiastic about the future and helps to realize that big dreams are much closer than they appear.

In this exercise, you will write a list of things you secretly want to do in your life. Those wishes and desires are something you are very passionate about but can be buried deep within. You might have never shared those with anyone (or yourself) and it is time to let them out.

The exercise consists of two parts: the crazy idea and the small challenge.

The Crazy Idea

For the first part of the exercise, write a list of 50 big and scary ideas that you want to accomplish in your lifetime. It can be an adventure, a project, a physical accomplishment, or even a travel destination. Don't limit yourself by what is possible or not. Let your imagination flow and put the ideas on paper. Usually, the creative process starts only after the first 20 or so obvious ideas are out of the way, so stick with it. It will get more interesting as you dig deeper.

These big ideas have to be scary and audacious, but also something that sparks a passion. Ideally, it should feel intimidating, but be something you are actually interested in and can imagine yourself doing. Rowing across the Atlantic Ocean, cycling from Europe to Asia, running the historical route 66. Whatever makes you inspired.

You can use the following questions to help you brainstorm:

1. If the next year was your last on Earth, what would you want to do, try, accomplish?
2. If you won the lottery, where would you go and what would you do?
3. What childhood dreams do you still want to fulfill?
4. What have you always wanted to do but have not done yet?
5. What experiences do you want to have/feel?
6. If you had an upcoming high school reunion, what would you like to tell your former classmates you have accomplished?
7. If you were asked to do a keynote at a large conference (on a topic you're very passionate about), what story do you wish you could tell the audience?

The Small Challenge

As the second part of the exercise, choose one idea that speaks the most to you and think of 1–2 achievable small challenges you can set for yourself right now that would move you a little closer to fulfilling it. The purpose is to lay out the path and create a series of small wins that move the boundary of what's comfortable in relation to the big, scary, and audacious goal. You might not go on to chase it, but at least you would have tried to—the small challenge will serve as a stepping stone to grow, instead of being paralyzed by fear.

This small challenge can be anything that is uncomfortable, but with dedication and focus, it is attainable. A self-supported multi-day hiking trip, a long-distance bike tour, an open water swim race, anything to get you started in the direction of your passion.

For example, someone with the crazy idea to climb mount Everest can set his or her first challenge to be finishing a marathon or completing a multi-day mountain hike. Training for either of these events will start developing the endurance and resilience needed for the big ascent. As the next challenge, that person might take it further and attempt the Everest challenge on a smaller mountain, covering the altitude of Mount Everest by going up and down within one or multiple days.

Besides acting as milestones, these smaller challenges help you to understand whether the big and crazy idea is indeed something that interests you or it is someone else's interest that the external world places on you.

BUILDING A CHARACTER

They say a dream come true reveals itself very slowly, but then all at once. That's because dreams are not linear. It takes a lot of effort to generate momentum and only once the pendulum is moving do things start to shape up and there is something to celebrate. Every so-called overnight success is built upon hours of consistent practice and, inevitably, failures.

Lack of immediate results, especially when we start something, often creates doubts and concerns. It does not help if a person has had negative experiences in the past that still impact his or her decisions. *'I've been running for a month already, but I'm not getting any faster. Yesterday I felt pain in my knee—will I be able to go on that skiing trip?'* But striving for results, being an overachiever, or burning to win at something is not a bad thing. The question is how people handle doubts, defeats, and failures.

Many athletes choose ignorance. They compartmentalize setbacks that they had in racing, training, or their personal life and store them somewhere deep inside. They don't work through what went wrong or take action to learn and improve. As a result, those negative experiences pile up and once they reach a certain threshold, it gets increasingly harder to break through them as they stack up and form an army. That threshold is often when an injury happens, or athletes develop certain pain and decide to stop training. The more times that knee hurts, the more an athlete confirms his or her belief about becoming too old.

In order to win at something, we first need to visualize victory. And that includes accepting that we are not perfect and need to consistently change. For athletes who tend to be ambitious by nature, it can be really hard to develop such humility and leave the ego aside, which is why denial in favor of being courageous is the most common practice. However, it is resilience that helps them to stay patient, quiet down concerns and keep putting the effort in.

It's healthy and perfectly normal to have a little bit of doubt—that's how we make progress and stay in touch with reality. Yes, our failures impact our life, but our resilience defines which direction. While some people carry their shortcomings on their backs as extra weight, others use them to create stepping stones and move up. We cannot fail in life—we can only fall short of the expectations we have put on ourselves. It is not a dead-end situation and definitely not a failure. Instead, it's an opportunity—to learn, to try again, to pivot, to change perspective and, ultimately, to grow. This opportunity is a precursor for faith and perseverance to go after our dreams even when things do not seem to work out.

Just like the Circle of Life, resilience is rooted in the character attributes, so to build confidence and persistence, we first need to understand who we are as individuals. In particular, understand that there are three driving forces which shape our unique personality and the ability to persevere: things we are interested in (passion), the cause we are following (purpose), and the principles we stick to (values and standards).

PASSION

We live in a world dominated by social norms, opinions, advertisement and peer pressure. Sometimes all of it makes sense and helps us advance our lives, but other times the external message is so "loud" that individuals are pushed to accept something that's not in their best interest. Like spending $300 on a pair of performance running shoes every so often (because professionals and influencers do that), instead of hiring a coach for a few months.

In a way, it is easier to follow someone else's footsteps than to do the things that matter to us. When there are rules, norms, or examples, there is also a clear set of instructions on what to do. There's nothing wrong with this approach, but it means that we are living someone else's life—not our own. It also becomes hard to realize our dreams and aspirations when we are trying to fit into standards defined by someone else.

Some athletes are prisoners of choice—they choose a sport and that becomes the lane they stick to or even define themselves by. '*I'm a runner, I'm a kayaker, I'm a gymnast.*' Yes, we are an ambitious bunch and we do want to get better, but the world is much wider than just that one lane. A good athlete is well-rounded and is able to take up any challenge—be it running a marathon, completing an adventure race, or going on a multi-day trek. We have the gift of fitness, why not use it to expand our horizons and make the most of our lives? It is a much wider definition of testing yourself and living up to your potential than simply beating a certain time in a marathon.

Knowing who we are, what we stand for, and owning it, takes courage and starts with not following the crowd. Our inner voice always knows what's best for us, which is why doing things that matter to us brings more joy than fitting in with the rest of the world. This is where passion steps in. It is the first of the forces that shape our character, and one that creates the initial spark to step out of the lane and begin moving in a new direction.

Finding that spark might come easy to some and very hard to others, depending on how open we are to testing ourselves and learning something new. In a way, it requires that we face our fears and are willing to let go of some degree of certainty and comfort, to make mistakes, look silly, or even miss out on something. It's all part of the process. A direct route is not always the best one, even if we don't see it right away. Often, we realize what our goals and dreams are only during the process.

As they say, you can only steer a moving ship, thus, the best way to find your calling is to first take any step and then pivot as you go. It is what the filmmaker Casey Neistat calls the Tarzan Method. Imagine you are on one side of the jungle and all your dreams and aspirations are on another side—in between there are just a bunch of trees and impenetrable bushes. To get across, you need to grab a liana, summon your courage and swing (like a Tarzan) to the next tree. It might not be a straight line, but it will get you closer to the other side. From there, you grab onto the next liana and swing further, which might take you a little off course, but still a little closer to where you are going. Finding passion is a continuous process of grabbing different lianas and, as you make your way through the jungle like a Tarzan, you sharpen your focus and discover what it is that drives you.

It might seem like that there is a straight line, an obvious path to reach a goal or fulfil a dream, but it is often an illusion created by the expectation of quick results. Life tends to take unexpected turns and in general does its best to derail us on the way to our dreams. In those low moments, we tend to think that we are not moving in the right direction or making any progress at all. However, when we look back, all the lessons we learned and experiences we built as a result of what happened, helped us to discover what we truly desire. All that we needed was courage to begin—to grab that next liana.

Doing something that sparks passion or brings joy is a great way to generate energy and positive motivation. So, make sure you have fun on a daily basis—both with others and by yourself. What we feel about the experience becomes the experience itself, so it is important to preserve playfulness which gives life its colors.

If you enjoy the process more than you enjoy the result—you are in a good place in life.

Doing something that we do not enjoy and relying on willpower to get us through the day is a recipe for disaster. Resilient athletes enjoy the process of pushing themselves to get better and learning where the limits are. As a result, they enjoy the training process more than they do the competition, which is why they are able to stay in the game for so long.

Step out of your current lane for a moment and look around. What are the things that interest you, but you held back from attempting for some reason? Those crazy and scary adventures you put on your bucket list in the previous exercise—was there a similar theme among those? In what way do those adventures inspire and drive you? And, more importantly, for what purpose?

STRATEGY: VISUAL CUES

How do we generate motivation and carry us through the rainy day runs, early morning workouts, or just going to the gym after work? By focusing on the intent, not the training or the activity itself.

First of all, imagine yourself at the end destination. What are you training for? Finishing a marathon? Becoming a Baywatch lifeguard? Or traveling to China to practice kung-fu? Picture it, feel it and, most importantly, focus on it. That mental picture will serve as a vision, so make it so vivid that you can describe anything about the experience of accomplishing the goal even when woken up in the middle of the night (i.e., sounds, smells, emotions, feelings, thoughts).

Next, ask yourself: Why does it matter to me? What is it that drives me? What do I want to achieve by accomplishing it? Answers to these questions won't reveal a deeper purpose, but they will help you to get closer and uncover the intent.

Finally, write down the current goal and intent behind it in a clear and short phrase and put it somewhere prominent, so you can see it all the time. Make sure you see this visual cue first thing in the morning so that you will start the day with a clear focus in mind. When you are feeling down, don't think of daunting exercises that you have to do. Instead, think of the vision you created, and the end result you will celebrate.

For example, if you are training to complete your first Ironman triathlon, your vision and intent might be I am training to become an Ironman. Obstacles and setbacks don't break me—they drive me.

We are more likely to succeed when we know where we are going. A vision has the power to guide us forward and help us to stay on track without any extra willpower. It's like New Year's resolutions—before we have them, we don't see the result, and we will not stick to the resolution for long.

PURPOSE

As a society, we have developed into a culture that glorifies hustle. It seems like there should always be something that we could or should be doing to optimize our life and deliver more in every area. Train more, finish the slides for the presentation next week, get groceries, or even meet with friends. With such a fast pace of everyday life and the amount of action points, it is easy to get overwhelmed and have a feeling as if we are falling behind. Not to mention that being fulfilled in life gets really hard when we do not feel the stable ground under our feet.

The demise of New Year's resolutions that happens every spring perfectly embodies the fragility of the hustle trend. In the first week of January, millions of people generate energy and excitement, as they reflect on what they want and set goals for the upcoming year. They are full of passion to bring change into their lives, and often they are quite consistent in it—exercising frequently, eating nutritious meals, drawing, learning to play a musical instrument and even reorganizing their lives. However, then there is that bump on the road that creates a crack in the plan—a night out with friends, a stressful day at work, an argument with a loved one, or just staying up late and missing the beauty sleep. Lo and behold, come March, the initial spark is gone and what's left is the harsh reality of how difficult it is to make good habits stick and how much time and effort is required to realize your dreams.

Nonetheless, we are often on the lookout for quick wins and ways to get things done faster—especially in the health and fitness area. Ten tips to lose body fat, four-week programs to boost strength gains and, of course, unlimited clues to live a happier and more fulfilling life. Most of the advice out there is indeed handy, but it is compressed into bite-sized chunks with the intent to grab attention and get the person started. In a way, to produce the New Year's resolution effect—ignite a spark and show direction. However, to continue with any practice, we need a more permanent solution than that. One of which will carry us through ups and downs, energize us and provide motivation to continue no matter how bumpy the path is. That solution is highly individual, yet the same for everyone. It is called a purpose.

There are days when we are so emotionally or physically tired that we do not want to wake up early, go on that 2-hour-long run, or prepare a nutritious meal. Such difficulties are nothing more than a test of our intention. Like a rite of passage, these mental hurdles are part of growing stronger and more resilient. Hard patches come up in our daily life, just like they do when running a marathon. **And we can face them like we would in a race: just focus on why we are doing it and simply keep putting one foot in front of the other.** In fact, that's something that Olympic middle-distance runner, Alexi Pappas, refers to as the rule of thirds.[1]

According to the rule, days when we are not feeling our best are just part of the process of chasing a dream or a hefty goal. In essence, we should expect to feel great one third of the time, feel normal one third of the time and feel bad one third of the time. When the ratio is off, we need to look at changing things. To put it into training perspective, if workouts feel easy or we feel great too often, maybe we are not challenging ourselves enough. On the other hand, if we are tired and lacking energy, frequently it can be a signal that we are pushing ourselves a little too hard and risk getting overtrained or burned out. More importantly, when there is a reason beyond just chasing endorphins, we do not abandon training. We show up for the good and bad days.

That last third seems like a lot of challenges that a person has to go through while chasing a dream. But the human body can sustain tremendous amounts of pressure if the purpose is strong. Sleep deprivation, hunger, cold—we have the ability to quiet down even such primal instincts simply by switching the focus from how we feel to how it makes us stronger.

Purpose is the second force that shapes personality and when we know ours, we feel that there is meaning behind what we do. It is something we love and enjoy, it pushes us out

---

1   In reference to Alexi Pappas's book "Bravery: Chasing Dreams, Befriending Pain, and Other Big Ideas"

of our comfort zone and forces us to grow, and it is something that is beyond just ourselves. Hence, there are three ingredients that form a strong purpose:

Purpose = passion + growth + contribution

You can call this the theme that we want our life to be about. The cause that we believe in so much that we put it at the core of everything we do. It is not always painless to stick to, but well worth it—a higher purpose consistently pushes us to do the uncomfortable and grow. People who don't have a higher purpose often find themselves following trends, running in circles and doing more of what they are already doing without challenging themselves enough. Have you ever thought about what you want your life to be about? What really matters to you?

A lot of training and racing involves connecting with ourselves—our potential, performance, and the present moment. In the spirit of competitiveness, that connection is often focused on tangible results. Beating a personal best, building more muscle, or dropping more fat, that's just how athletes are wired. However, performance will eventually decline, and we want to continue on the path to becoming the best version of ourselves indefinitely. That includes not using sports to run away from problems and hide from the reality of life, but to run towards something bigger. A cause that is worth devoting our time to—day in and day out.

While the quest for peak performance is significantly about an individual—results, records, and medals—the quest of life is all about purpose and meaning.

Finding a cause that's meaningful requires us to look deep within and reconnect with our essence. Our mind will always focus on problems, speak up and find reasons for why things will not work out. Once we connect with the heart and soul, discover what brings us fulfillment, and use it to guide us, that is when we can become fully committed to the task instead of merely interested. In fact, when we accomplish something and feel like it is not enough, that is the world helping us to continue to grow. It means that the goal we set for ourselves is just that, a goal. As hefty as it might be, it is not a mountain to climb, but rather a peak to be traversed on a journey to something more substantial.

Purpose is a powerful tool that guides companies through hard times, and it is even more powerful for individuals. The right cause motivates us no matter what the environment is or what people say. With that in mind, we are able to turn any negativity and doubt into the rocket fuel that will power us through.

To help an individual power through adversity, a strong purpose has to be bigger than just one race or one achievement. The stronger it is, the better he or she can navigate the inevitable bumps on the road. Otherwise, it is just a passion—a spark that gives direction but does not carry much energy. The excitement of the upcoming race will guide an athlete through the workouts to prepare for the distance but will subside as soon as the race is over. However, when a goal is a part of a bigger purpose, it will force us to grow consistently—not peak for one experience—and always guide us to the next step. For example, being fit and healthy gives us the energy and the ability to be adventurous and try new things.

Besides that, purpose should also span beyond ourselves to survive the test of time. When we focus on what we want, we never get past our own problems—unlimited needs, concerns, and fears. However, when we turn the tables around and think "how we can be of service and contribute to the lives of others," that's where the magic starts to happen. Focusing on giving more helps us to adopt a more strategic perspective and use our strengths instead of fixating on what's holding us back. Be it coaching, creating a community or just being a mentor to the younger generation—whatever it takes to move the spotlight away from us.

In fact, growth and contribution are the only two human needs that cannot be fully met. We can fulfill the need for certainty, significance, entertainment, and accomplishments, but we cannot fully grow or contribute to others' lives enough. Those two needs are the backbone of achieving our full potential and, therefore, are great stimuli to guide us beyond the limits we unintentionally set for ourselves. There is little that tests and pushes the limits more than an ultra-endurance adventure.

PERSONAL STANDARDS

The Ironman triathlon is considered the single toughest one-day sporting event in the world. It's a 2.4-mile (3.8K) swim, 112-mile (180K) bike ride and a full 26.2-mile (42.2K) marathon—all in one go. The race starts shortly before 7AM and whoever crosses the finish line before midnight is considered an Ironman. Completing such an endurance challenge is a process of discovering what you are really made of but is also excruciatingly difficult. Besides physical exhaustion, it is essentially a very long and tedious (for some up to 17 hours) conversation with yourself.

Strength, endurance, and resilience are not only physical attributes. How fast a person runs or what distance he or she can cover might be the deciding factor in a race when everything goes right—an ideal scenario. But a long-distance race (let alone an ultra-endurance one) is hardly ever perfect. A lot can happen over the course of a 10+ hour day—goggles fogged or slipped, a flat tire, knee pain, an upset stomach, muscle cramps, and so much more. Which is why being strong, enduring, and resilient is about how a person performs when everything goes wrong, whether he or she is able to consistently stand up after being knocked on the knees. In that sense, life is a lot like the Ironman triathlon. It is not about who is the fastest, but rather about who breaks down and slows down the least.

As much as they hurt and are inconvenient, setbacks and adversity are part of the training process—for a race and life in general. No matter how mentally strong we are, it is always uncomfortable to go through a challenging experience, especially because it is something we are never entirely ready for. The pandemic of 2020 was the best example for that—nobody was ready for the world to essentially halt for an entire year. The rules have changed. Isolation was something very few of us had experienced before. Plans we made and goals we set for our life had been interrupted. However, such challenges also provided the environment to practice the skill of resilience. A change like COVID-19 creates a huge opportunity for whoever is ready to do more, practice, gain the understanding, knowledge, skills, and inspiration needed to turn that experience around.

"I am not afraid of storms, for I am learning how to sail my ship."

— LOUISA MAY ALCOTT

We are not defined by what happens to us. We shape ourselves by choosing how we respond to events, whether we hide from adversity or step up and face it. Our personal standards, therefore, are the third force that shapes the character. Core values we hold ourselves to and principles we follow is what has the power to push us to go that extra mile, do more than required, and reach beyond what we can grab. These standards serve as the lighthouse for us and do not let us settle for anything below what we expect of ourselves.

Dreams and expectations alone don't move an athlete closer to his or her goals. Elite athletes get to the top of the sport not because of talents or natural gifts. They do so because they demand more of themselves than anyone expects, and act based on what they feel they are worth. Extraordinary outcomes come from extraordinary standards, and by identifying ourselves in a certain way and sticking with it against all odds, we eventually become the standard we hold ourselves to.

They say how we do anything is how we do everything. Those who have low standards are held by them in everything they do—when their priority is to avoid doing the hard thing or just to get something over with, it conditions the mind not to try as hard. This applies to a particular task, or any other activity. Low standards, therefore, prevent people from putting in more effort, going the extra mile, and trying their best.

However, this goes the other way as well—we can raise our standards by backing those with consistent practices. Stretching ourselves, committing to doing the uncomfortable, always trying our best, challenging ourselves in different ways, and even training in harsh conditions to become unbreakable. When we feel low on energy, that is the signal to keep going. The moment we want to give up or get distracted is an opportunity to break the pattern of sparing yourself and create a new one—of persevering. Top performers show up and look for ways to become 1% better every single day. So can we.

The bravest thing we can do in life is to try our best—at any point in time. It's scary to be vulnerable, to tell yourself I am worth it and shoot for the moon. It takes courage to take the responsibility into your own hands, accept the consequences and remove the option of purposefully failing, only to have an excuse for why things have not worked out. Taking that leap makes all the difference. Giving our best shot unconsciously raises our standards, creates an emotional connection and gives ourselves permission to achieve those extraordinary results we expect.

Good effort brings mediocre results because everyone else makes a good effort. Good results happen when we give our best. But when we go above and beyond, that's when we get exceptional results. Becoming a top performer is about consistently going the extra mile and winning that battle against your mind that urges you to stop. Some days it will be running one extra mile, other days it will be just showing up. Success will not always go as we hope or plan it to, but that's part of the deal. The practice of giving your best provides a launching pad,—an opportunity to become better. Every top performer started somewhere and settled for anything less than his or her best. The more we can challenge ourselves physically and mentally, the easier the racing experience will feel and the better prepared we will be for when things do not go so well.

Everyone who has achieved a lot in life will tell you that it wasn't an overnight success and required hard work and discipline. However, discipline does not mean to work hard or hustle. On their own these words don't mean a thing. Hustle and hard work have to be backed by a very high standard of not accepting anything less than personal excellence. If we want to become the best versions of ourselves, then that has to become our standard. Not once in a while, not when we feel like it, but every single day.

SNEAK PEEK: SHOW UP, KEEP UP AND REPEAT THE NEXT DAY

Every autumn during my competitive kayaking career, our training group would focus on aerobic base training. Since there was little daylight and time was tight on weekdays due to work or studies, our only option to add volume was on weekends. And so, we did. Two back-to-back long days—a three-hour-long session on Saturday and the same one on Sunday.

These sessions were very exhausting, and we couldn't fully adjust to them. In sprint kayaking, one race lasts anywhere from 30 seconds to just under 4 minutes, so three hours two days in a row was a stretch. It hurts to sit for that long, let alone to kayak. The unpredictable weather was always a factor—temperatures in November and December were barely above freezing and usually accompanied by a strong wind. And, on top of that, you had to keep up—we were typically a group of four and it was not a walk in the park, to say the least.

In terms of keeping up, kayaking is like cycling. It's easier when you are in a group, because you can use the wave that comes off another boat to save some energy, but once you fall off, it gets increasingly harder to carry on alone. If you are not near another boat and in the correct position, that same wave that worked for you will push you back instead.

The pace of those three-hour-long sessions was hard to maintain, especially in the first few weeks when the body was adjusting to the workload. But it was the company of like-minded individuals that pushed each of us to stay in the group, even when the mind screamed to slow down. It was hard for everyone, yet nobody was willing to give up—finishing the session in the leading group always brought a strong sense of accomplishment—not to mention that you would finish earlier. Ironically, the toughest part of training was not the workload, cold weather or exhaustion, but the realization on Saturday afternoon that even though you are really tired, you have to do the same thing the next day. That was the standard we held each other to—show up, give your best and don't let go when things get tough.

What I found outside of the professional athlete life is that standards generally are much lower. There's rarely one specific event that we work towards (like the World Championship of email sending), so we tend to cut ourselves some slack every now and then. Having more things to balance (work, family, etc.) means we have to make compromises and due to mental fatigue, sometimes that means taking the easy path. It's been a hard day at work, I'll run tomorrow morning. Maybe watching TV today isn't a bad idea—I'll be more productive tomorrow. I'm spending a lot of time on social media, but hey, who doesn't?

Such excuses are like a boomerang. They feel great in the moment and take the imminent pressure off, as we realize we're not obliged to do the hard thing. However, that pressure is required for growth. So, after a while, that boomerang returns with the realization that each excuse costs at least a day of effort and could have been put towards achieving a goal. When we set our own standards, we become resistant to such excuses and external opinions, which unblocks the path towards our goals.

Standard is not always the perfect result or perfectionism for that matter. Sometimes we need to play the cards we have been dealt. In my case, we could not affect the weather during those three-hour-long training sessions or ensure we were fresh and recovered for every single one of them, but giving our best in any situation is something we could do, so we accepted nothing less.

BALANCING THE THREE FORCES

Every athlete at some point secretly imagines him- or herself leading a race with nobody in sight. Or being atop the podium with minimum effort. An easy victory as a reward for the daily grind. But what is there to learn from easy? Not much. It's great to please the ego, of course, but from an experience standpoint there is little value. When things go horribly wrong, in my case it was the middle of the night during the kayak marathon, that's when we are truly put through a test and forced to face our character. With all its strengths and shortcomings.

I found endurance sports to be a perfect mechanism for self-discovery and transformation. A physical, emotional and, some might say spiritual, adventure to discover my authentic self. The longer the distance I was competing in, the deeper I had to reach to re-discover my passion, purpose, and personal standards. Mentally I was able to focus and "muscle" my way through a few minutes of maximum effort without a hitch, but resilience is something you cannot fake for 10+ hours in a narrow boat in the middle of the night. Eventually, you will get to that dark place where you have to face your inner demons.

When I think about that overnight adventure, I feel thankful for the experience. The memory of it makes me feel more alive than hundreds of shorter races I did. And while I am grateful for those as well, there was little purpose behind them, aside from maximizing what my body is able to deliver within a span of just under four minutes. At some point, professional kayaking even became mentally destructive because I got obsessed with it and reluctant to try new things. The challenge served as an opportunity to step back and get some perspective on the small box I found myself in.

When I finished that overnight kayak marathon, I got a feeling that I had accomplished something more substantial than in any other race, even though I didn't get a medal. Only a finisher T-shirt and a sticker for 4th place. Nonetheless, I felt as if I stepped on the path to self-discovery and unlocked a new level. In my head, it was no longer about becoming uber-fit for one race that I did a hundred times but becoming fit for life with all its adventures. So, after sleeping for 20 hours straight, I grew more excited about the quality I will bring to my training with this new purpose. And, more importantly, in this perspective I was (and still am) yet to tap into my true potential.

Truth is, I was not the only athlete who struggled with something and didn't know what it was. So many good athletes drop training because they lose the spark. They are concerned that the glory days have passed and that exhilarating feeling of immersing yourself in the moment will not happen again. However, this is not the case. Becoming the best version of ourselves is an ongoing journey and sometimes we need to make a shift to stay on track. Discover the passion again—one that lights us up and makes us forget about the rest of the world. Take it to the next level and craft a bigger purpose—whatever brings value to us and others. Go on an inside journey to discover who we are and what we stand for.

The challenge—or rather beauty—of life is that it is not about achieving one single goal. Otherwise, all the top performers would be happy and fulfilled. On the contrary, happiness spans all areas of life and is always a combination of various factors. When we overfocus on a single area we risk becoming unfulfilled in others, just like a workaholic who has a successful career that came at the expense of personal health and quality of relationships. We get better experiences when we are fit and well, not when we use all our energy on training and then suffer from feeling unfulfilled in other areas (career, relationships, emotional, financial). Professional sports careers will eventually end. We will complete that marathon, but what happens next? Are we preparing ourselves for the next season of our life? Or are we living for the moment?

Everyone has his or her own recipe for finding fulfillment, but it comes down to paying equal attention to every force that shapes the character—passion, purpose, and standards. Resilient athletes have all these three forces in balance, and they are as motivated to start something as they are to push through and go the extra mile to become the best version of themselves.

A resilient athlete is first and foremost someone who is focused on the future and long-term. He or she invests in physical and emotional health and prioritizes growth over immediate results. Naturally, such a wide perspective helps to rebound quicker, to use failures as stepping stones and not let the past define the future. A resilient athlete is able to do so because he or she has developed a high level of self-awareness and knows what's important in the long-term. Thanks to high personal standards, he or she is committed to doing what is meaningful and not settling for the shortcut.

EXERCISE: DISCOVER YOUR PERSONAL POWER

Imagine this: you get up early, jump out of bed, excited for the day ahead. You are energized, enjoy whatever you do and do not hesitate to put the extra effort in. It doesn't feel difficult because the hours seem to zoom right by. How does that sound? Are you living this dream? Do you wake up excited?

There's a type of person who seem to radiate confidence and who we are therefore happy to spend time with. They're happy, relaxed, naturally charismatic, confident and seem to know what they want in life. They are magnetic without being "too much." Listening to them speak, you feel as though you would gladly follow them to the ends of the earth. And they might even leave you thinking "wow, I wish I could be like them!"

These people aren't unicorns and were not born with unnatural abilities to get everything right in life. They are regular people who have discovered their "personal power" and learned to govern it. The exercise below will help you find yours and start building a foundation for that state of absolute confidence.

Discovering personal power is about paying equal attention to the three forces that shape the character—passion, purpose, and standards.

Step 1: Find Passion to Create a Spark

The idea of finding passion can sound daunting…especially when you are surrounded by people on social media who seem to have it all figured out and "just know" what they want to do for the rest of their lives. Rather than focusing on what everyone else is doing, adopt a curious attitude about life. Then passion will naturally unfold before you. Let your intuition guide you towards those options and activities that are perhaps less obvious, but you always wanted to try. It might seem irrelevant or impractical but trust yourself: you are drawn to these things for a reason.

For some, that spark might come as a result of finishing a race. For others it can appear during one of the exciting adventures that being in great shape enables (surf camps, trekking adventures, kayaking trips, etc.). It can be as simple as joining a community to enjoy the company while exercising. Whatever intrigues you.

Close your eyes and imagine everything you ever wanted. Imagine vividly, as if you already have it and ask yourself honestly—what does perfect look like to me? Use the questions below to help you get started. Do not reject an idea right away if it sounds silly. We do this all the time to avoid thinking about specifics because they are scary. They define not only what you want, but the parameters of failure if you do not get them. Instead, explore the idea fully and find the underlying reason why you find it intriguing.

- What do I love to do?
- What would my ideal day look like if I was doing what I love?
- What interests have I had in the last few years that intrigue me and I might consider trying?
- What do I spend a lot of time reading about when I should be doing other things?
- What are some childhood interests or dreams that I never was able to explore fully, but still find intriguing?
- What skills or talents do I have that I am passionate about using?

Write down whatever comes to mind, a free flow of ideas. The same way you did when creating a bucket list, but this time once you review your brainstorm, think critically about the triggers. What draws you towards those outcomes? Why do you want to engage in a certain activity? Is that a universal trigger you can replicate in a different area? These underlying desires are where passion originates.

For someone who loves to run, it can be about self-discovery and the freedom running provides. It feels extraordinary to be reaching for the limit and liberating to feel immersed in the moment. To be fully present and focus on the process (not the outcome) and have room to grow. Can this growth and freedom be created in other areas as well, like work or family, and trigger a passion?

Step 2: Create a Purpose That Helps to Push Through the Hard Bits

The way to navigate through periods of low morale is to develop an exciting "why am I doing it?" A vision you can turn to in times of doubt. Few people actually take the time to think about what they want their life to be about and, therefore, struggle to find the reason to continue when a certain level of success has been reached. Being honest with yourself about your "why" and framing it as something that drives you (not pushes you) is what makes the difference between taking action and leaving it for tomorrow.

Remember the formula **Purpose = Passion + Growth + Contribution**. Have you ever thought about what really matters to you, besides personal enjoyment? What makes you feel fulfilled, and you would like to have more of? These are some of the hardest questions to answer truthfully, but those answers reveal the purpose that can help guide your everyday life. When you know what your life is about, you can ask yourself whether what you do on a daily basis contributes to your purpose. If not, take gradual steps to change it for the better.

Use the questions below and reflect on what's meaningful to you:

- What areas of my current life are working well for me? What do I find fulfilling, meaningful and important about them?
- Why do I want my ideal future (for other reasons than personal enjoyment)?
- What situations make me feel fulfilled, what do I do and who am I with?
- What do I enjoy learning about?
- If I knew I was going to die one year from today, what would I do and how would I want to be remembered?
- If money wasn't an issue, what would I do with my life?
- How am I going to save the world?
- What do I love doing that also helps others?

Purpose is the intersection between what sparks passion for you, what makes you grow and where you can contribute. Use the passion you have discovered in the previous step and look for a purpose behind it. What is it in those activities that would stimulate you to grow? How can you make it not about yourself? Fill in the blanks below to help you define a meaningful cause:

I can't wait to get out of bed, and I could stay up all night to do _____. It makes me a better person because _____. It helps others because _____.

Step 3: Establish Values and Standards to Stay Accountable

The final step is to get a clear understanding of yourself—what you stand for and what is the most important thing to you. That knowledge keeps you grounded in life, gives you confidence to follow your own path, and prevents you from falling into the trap of making others happy. When you truly understand what kind of a person you are and what you stand for, you will be able to bring the state of absolute certainty and courage into your actions and tell yourself, '*I will find a way, or I will make a way.*'

Core values power our standards—they make us who we are and help us make decisions that are right for us. By defining what your core values are, you will be in a better position to set goals that will allow you to stay true to your personal ethics, as well as assist in your growth as a person. So, find whatever drives you, reconnect with it and stay true to it.

For example: what is it about sports that you're so passionate about? Is it the quest for excellence and consistently pushing yourself to get better? Or is it self-discipline and befriending pain and discomfort for the purpose of delayed gratification? Once you notice values attached to the activity, you can bring those to whatever you do and, therefore, bring that activity to a whole new level.

Take a few moments to think about what kind of person you aim to become and what are the driving forces for you? Consider all the things that make you feel like you. What do you truly value in those? Write down the core values that are important to you. Examples include integrity, respect, family, work ethic, sense of humor.

Next, think of the people with characters you look up to the most, your role models. Those can be either from your inner circle or any public figure (real or imagined, alive or dead)—whoever inspires you. What are the behaviors that you look up to? What principles and values drive those behaviors?

Finally, answer the following questions to determine what your standards need to be:

- How does my life currently reflect values that are important to me (in every area)?
- What has to change for me to live the life that reflects these values?
- What standards do I need to develop for myself to live that life?
- What can I no longer accept if I want to succeed?
- What MUST I do to get what I want (instead of SHOULD)?

EMOTIONAL FITNESS

There is one thing I always come back to throughout my life: water, in all of its forms. I used to swim when I was in primary school. Then it was kayaking through high school and university. And after that, it was open water swimming in triathlons. For as long as I can remember I was always fascinated by the idea of learning to surf. Something about the process sparks my imagination and I can see many parallels with life in it.

Surfing is very humbling. Especially when you are first learning, a lot of the time you are not even on the board: you are in the process of getting up on it or falling off of it. Every ride ends in the water whether you like it or not, so you need to find energy and courage every time to get up and paddle back to the lineup while navigating crashing waves. For a beginner, this process is very exhausting, but with every wipeout, you learn how not to do things. My first surf camp was a whirlwind adventure in the most literal way, as I was thrown around by every wave. However, I also learned that once you consider it a necessary practice, you don't hesitate to get back up. By trying as much as possible you get the opportunity to analyze what you did wrong and improve further.

Even when you do get good, it doesn't mean you've made it. Surfing requires patience and accepting the fact that conditions in the ocean always change. You can be as ready as possible, but you won't know for sure how big the wave will come, where it will peak compared to where you are, or even in which direction the wind will change. No two waves are exactly the same, so you cannot become very attached to certain expectations. Otherwise, you will always feel anxious that things are not going according to plan. The ocean is always moving and has its own agenda, and the best surfer is the one who takes what the situation can offer and has the most fun.

Whether we like it or not, things always change in life. Often in a very unexpected ways and at the last minute. Traffic jams take place when we are in a hurry, work meetings run late when we absolutely have to get off work earlier, races get cancelled and travel plans fall apart. The world is not going to stop changing—that's what keeps it alive. The question is are we going to stress about everything going on around us? Or will we learn to let it go and live life on our own terms despite it all?

Our experience of life is shaped by the emotional states we go through in response to certain events, activities, and situations. Happiness, sadness, joy, frustration, love—these are just a few examples of how we might feel about whatever happens to or around us. It is important to remember that how we feel is nothing more than a state of mind created by our nervous system. If it's something that originates in our head, only we have the power to control it and impact our lives. Nobody else.

We can have all the strength, skills, talent, and preparation in the world, but if we are not able to put emotions aside and focus on the task at hand when it matters, we will succumb to pressure—be it internal (doubts and fear) or external (opinions and expectations). **A resilient athlete is not only physiologically strong and enduring, but has also learned to use, manage and direct emotions.** Such capacity is what gets people through the hard days, weeks, months or even years. There is nothing that can stop a person who is emotionally unshakable. No matter what others think or how crazy things are, he or she remains calm, determined and focused.

Each of us has had certain experiences in life that subconsciously started to define our response to what happens. People who are able to cure their emotional pain will not be as affected by external events as those who bear the weight of such baggage. They won't be stopped by thinking *what if* and instead will tackle setbacks as they come—with confidence. Such people are still open for opinions, feedback, and new ideas, but don't take them personally. Instead, they thrive on them.

It's called emotional fitness because this capacity to quiet down the noise of the world and focus on what's important for us is something that can be trained. Much like physical fitness, sustaining the skill to clear your mind and control your emotional response requires practice. To become mentally strong and resilient against stressful situations, we must condition our mind with the same effort that we condition our muscles.

When we stop training our muscles, they atrophy. When we stop strengthening our mind, it goes back to low emotional fitness.

The absence of such focus makes the training process less effective. In particular, athletes who lack self-control are more likely to:

- Think about something else during sessions.
- Spend more time talking (or using social media) than training.
- Do something that interferes with the quality of training (poor sleep quality, unhealthy diet, staying out late and partying).
- Skip sessions altogether.

Many talented athletes struggle in their late teens and stop training because there are many distractions that take the attention away from training which requires more discipline and consistency than ever.

Emotional fitness provides a strong backbone that a person can lean on when things get rough or uncertain. It generates confidence that lets an athlete say to him or herself, '*Whatever happens, I can handle it*.' Being emotionally resilient means there is nothing that can negatively affect a decision or behavior in the moment because there is no emotional attachment to it. It's one of the most important factors to overcome obstacles in life, because it helps us to adapt to circumstances and always choose the most optimal course of action.

EMBRACING CHANGE

Change is an integral part of our life. We transform from cuddly bundles of joy into individuals with interests and opinions that constantly evolve. And so does the world around us. Population grows, technology advances, new discoveries are being made—everything has an impact on the way we live our lives.

However, change is not an easy thing to befriend because of the stormy weather of uncertainty it brings along. A lot of people do not step out into the unknown and would much rather hang out in a comfort bubble waiting for the waves to calm down. While this cautious approach is safer, in the longer term it ends up limiting our potential.

It's a myth that we need the outside world to be OK for us to be OK. An excuse we subconsciously tell ourselves to be able to pause when we feel like we are not in control or the pace of the world is too fast. We live in times when everything can change in an instant and one year from now our life will be different. The question is how different. Will it be the life that ends up happening or the one we choose to live? We can resist change, be defensive, stay on the sidelines and, eventually, fall behind. Or, we can be proactive instead, accept the situation, and look for ways to grow along with the change.

The progress we make in life is not a given. It's subject to how willing we are to go through pain and discomfort. **Change can be painful, but just like muscle growth requires pain, change is necessary for our growth as individuals.** We don't know what we don't know, so if we are not changing, we have no other way to expand our perspective and live up to our full potential. If we want to become the best versions of ourselves, we need to constantly reinvent and look for ways to get better.

I found that switching from professional kayaking to long-distance triathlons embodies the concept of embracing change to me. Making a shift like that and stepping away from what I thought I wanted for close to 15 years was a hard decision, but it made me stronger and more confident as an athlete. It was just what I needed to grow my perspective and avoid becoming tied to one discipline and one way of living. Triathlon was interesting and challenging enough to try out, but it was the shift itself that pushed the limits of what I am comfortable with and was the driving force behind my consistent progress.

The truth is the world will not wait for us to be ready for it. If we do not keep up, life will force us to by giving us a grueling test. On the bright side, whoever accepts the fact that things can always change and welcomes the uncertainty (instead of stressing about it), will find that fear evaporates. When we think of ourselves as experimenters and adopt a learning mindset towards outcomes, we will focus on learning something that will get us closer to our desired results and not get stuck fixating on whether or not we will get the result we want.

In surfing, finding peace in conditions of constant change is a crucial part of the process. We might expect to have the ride of our lives, but the ocean usually has its own agenda. The waves might be too big or too small. The wind can be blowing too hard making waves unrideable. There can be current, rain or even too many other surfers. Instead of being frustrated at not having the desired experience, a much healthier approach is to treat it as a learning process. Remove any expectations and have more fun, that's what surfing is about.

Having a learner's mindset doesn't mean rushing into things and ignoring adversity—leaders do anticipate and prepare themselves for what might happen. Which is why when training for a race, it's important to consider what hurdles you might encounter (physical or mental) and prepare accordingly. If it's heat, work to adapt yourself to handle hot conditions better. If it's a hilly race, practice running uphill and downhill. If it's going to be wet, practice in the rain. Don't get paralyzed by the fear of the unknown, adjust your expectations and play the cards you're dealt.

We cannot always control what happens in a race (or in life), but we can control our response to it by means of emotional fitness. You will find the framework to condition your mind in the exercise section of this chapter, but for it to be effective it's important to develop the courage to push against the hopelessness and stay ahead of the change. Doing so helps to find comfort in the unknown but requires a high degree of self-awareness.

SELF-AWARENESS

Feelings and emotions add color and flavor to life. Without those things, every day would be the same and every event, activity or experience would be meaningless. However, in some situations, emotions get the better of us. Let's be honest, we have all had moments when we lost our temper, said something we shouldn't have or did something we later regret. After all, we are humans, not robots, and unless we pay close attention, it is very hard to realize what's happening until we are too far down the "emotional rabbit hole" to change it.

These low moments that are created by negative emotional states are like micro-injuries to our character. If left untreated, they tend to repeat themselves and form into specific patterns depending on the situations they arise in. As we get into the habit of giving in to negative emotional states, those small injuries stack up and start to drag our energy down. Anger. Frustration. Exhaustion. Burnout. All of this is caused by emotional fatigue as a result of stress.

So, in a way, we can injure ourselves by means of consistent negative experiences, just like we can injure any other part of our body as a result of overuse and insufficient recovery. While such emotional injuries are not so visible in a high-paced environment of competitive sports, that doesn't mean they are not there. **Every time an athlete is unable to focus, has a hard time coping with pressure or is generally feeling restless, there's a reason for that.** Maybe it's connected to a negative experience that occurred in a race. Or as a result of consistently not meeting expectations. Maybe it is caused by a stressful situation that occurred a long time ago, but never processed. Either way, we need to let it heal just like any other injury—recovery is equally important for both physical and emotional wellness.

In sports, there is a saying: Stress + Rest = Progress. If we want to build our emotional fitness and become more resilient to external factors, we have to give ourselves enough rest to process the events and activities that caused us stress. Just like in training, it is active rest that promotes emotional recovery—processing what has happened and learning to deal with hard emotional moments better so that they affect you less.

The starting point of any self-development journey is through awareness. In the case of building emotional resilience, it is first recognizing how we feel (angry, anxious, fearful, ashamed, or otherwise draining our energy) and which events or situations make us feel that way. How do I currently feel about myself? Is there any tension? What causes me to feel stressed, anxious, angry, or otherwise not at my best? It helps to have a support network to discuss it with, someone to ask for feedback, or at least to use a journal and record thoughts in private. Often, recognizing the thought patterns that occur inside our head helps us reevaluate how important those are and, therefore, reduce the weight we carry on our shoulders.

Our habits and lifestyle are the reflection of our emotional state and a logical place to begin digging for evidence. Training, sleep, diet, and even the way we interact and communicate is affected by how we process emotions and regulate ourselves. In fact, the training process is a particularly visual example of it. Many amateur athletes use sport as a mechanism to deal with stress and training sessions as a way to unload pressure. Ironically, this leads to burnout or overtraining because such training sessions become too intense and often unstructured. More experienced athletes also suffer from overtraining and burnout, but it typically comes from the fear of "falling behind." They lack confidence to listen to their body and its needs, so they push the body too hard, train through fatigue or even train twice a day, not because the body needs it, but because everyone else does it.

Give yourself some time to slow down and reflect on how your lifestyle supports or drains you. Look for the following red flags to help discover patterns:

- Being easily irritable or edgy. Frustration, even over small matters.
- Consistent feelings of sadness, melancholy, emptiness, or hopelessness.
- Inability to concentrate.
- Sleep disturbances, including insomnia or sleeping too much.
- Increased awareness of aches and pains.
- Changes in appetite and eating (including cravings).
- Overtraining, injuries, burnout, plateaus.
- Doubts and loss of self-esteem. Loss of interest in most or all normal activities.

Competitive nature often doesn't let athletes admit that they have flaws. Believing we are invincible just feels so much better. However, if we don't engage in self-reflection, it doesn't mean we do not have problems, we are just choosing to ignore them. Everyone has an area or two where he or she can put more effort in. And as much as bringing it to the personal spotlight can be painful (be it personal or external feedback), becoming aware of personal shortcomings is crucial to becoming better.

Think of self-reflection as bloodwork, a test for how well the system is running. If athletes do not get their bloodwork done on a consistent basis, that doesn't mean they don't have low iron or high cholesterol levels. It just means they haven't found out about it yet. Resilient athletes are able to consistently improve and grow stronger with age because they are humble. They accept flaws and defeat, which helps them to see clearly what the weak areas are that they have to develop.

After embracing change, self-reflection is the second step towards emotional fitness. Its aim is to establish a connection between actions, thoughts, and emotions. The final step is to learn to detach feelings from thoughts and actions to emotionally regulate.

EMOTIONAL REGULATION

Sometimes our actions (or inactions) in life are based out of fear and not necessarily passion. Fear of failure. Fear of rejection. Fear of being judged. '*What if something doesn't work out? How would it make me look? What if they don't like me?*' We develop these fears because we try to avoid pain associated with them. But it is not the fear itself that matters, but our emotional response to it. Response determines the quality of decisions we make and actions we take, which, eventually, impacts beliefs about our ambitions and potential (as per the Circle of Life).

Imagine hiring a CEO for your life whose task would be to ensure everything is in place for long-term success. Craft a big and meaningful purpose. Organize the lifestyle to get as much energy as possible. Motivate every morning to live the day with passion. Would you want to hire someone who is afraid of taking action and concerned about his or her potential? Or would you choose someone who can get things done whatever the pressure? Everyone already has this personal CEO: it's our mind, the one that calls all the shots in life, and it develops depending on what we feed to it. If we focus on fear, we become more fearful. If we focus on courage, we become more courageous.

When we give in to fear, it paralyzes us and prevents us from taking any action. The truth is, we are all afraid of something. **Fear is a natural state and even has a purpose: to protect us from potential danger and help us survive.** It has tremendous power to wake us up and force us to act; the question is how do we use that power? Do we choose to live life running away from pain or break the pattern once and set ourselves up for success going forward?

A disempowered way to live life is fear-based: reacting to events, following the trends, thinking as if everything is predetermined. Living with passion, on the other hand, is action-based and puts the control in the individual's hands. When we break the pattern of fear with action, that's when things start to shift, and we experience freedom and power over adversity.

So, get out of your comfort zone and bulletproof yourself. Face whatever the fear is and if your mind or body tells you today is not the day for something, that is the signal that you absolutely must do it. But don't complain; it's a destructive habit that only cultivates negative thought processes. Be grateful for the opportunity to better yourself. Think of all the things that made you who you are and appreciate how the experience you are going through will make you more resilient. You can't be fearful and grateful at the same time—gratefulness will edge fear out.

SNEAK PEEK: FACING THE FEAR OF MASS STARTS

When I started kayaking in my early teens, I used to be very afraid of competitions that included mass starts. The whole idea of tens (if not hundreds) of boats lining up each within an arms-length of another and charging forward the moment the gun goes off was terrifying to me. For several years I was nervous before such competitions and always positioned myself at the back, afraid of falling off the kayak and being run over. Ironically, that was what made me consistently fall in the cold water, because the waves of other boats were moving in all directions and balancing became close to impossible.

One year I decided I couldn't keep living like that. I was training hard, but due to my fear I had nothing to show for it—roughly half of the mass start races I had started by that point of time I did not finish. I felt like I had nothing to lose, so I positioned myself in the front row and started as hard as I could. To my surprise, after the first 500 meters there were only six of us going into the first turn—not much different than during a training session.

Every time we feel anxious or nervous before the race or event, it is the fear of the unknown that is taking over. *'What if something happens and I can't show my best? What if I do show my best, but it is average? What would others think of me?'* In moments like these it helps to distance yourself from the fact itself and consider the worst-case scenario. Play it out in your head beforehand and decide if it's something you can live with should it materialize.

For me, the worst-case scenario was that I would be out of the boat, in the cold water in wet clothes with lots of other boats moving fast nearby. Sounds scary, but I have been in that situation a few times before during training and am still alive, so there's hope. After all, I'm a decent swimmer, there's always a rescue boat nearby, and it's not even a given that I'm going to fall over. And just like that, the moment I started believing in myself and took action, every scary situation I imagined evaporated.

In its essence, mental strength is the ability to do what others won't. For athletes, that often is the deciding factor (in training or racing), as harsh conditions, setbacks and external pressure will impact an athlete's emotional state and prevent him or her from giving his best. But negative emotional states we find ourselves in—sadness, anxiousness, envy, etc.—are largely defined by our response to external stimuli. In other words, it is our thought processes that makes us nervous before a race, feel anxious when someone is rude to us, or feel sad when we hear bad news. Often, we cannot change or impact the situation we're in, but we sure can change our response to it.

Our actions and accomplishments trigger certain thoughts which make us feel a certain way—happy, sad, joyful, and so on. We can get attached to some of these feelings and focus on chasing a certain result to experience that feeling again. Win a race to feel significant. Go on a holiday to feel calm. Meet someone to feel loved. It is great to have a goal and chase endorphins, but this way we will always chase tangible things to experience a certain feeling. Run more marathons, build more muscle, please more people.

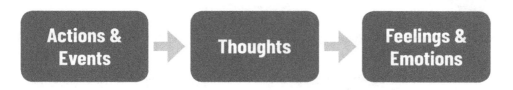

The process of emotional development. Actions change first, then thoughts, then feelings.

A more effective approach to controlling your emotional state is to learn to detach yourself from it and focus on what is best for you. We can't force feeling (or not feeling) a certain way or expect our feelings to change without doing something about it. Without the thought process, there is no basis for feelings and emotions to develop and without a triggering event there's nothing even to think about. So, our actions need to change first, then thoughts, and only then will our emotional state be different. In other words, we can control how we emotionally react to situations by taking action and changing the way we see events and situations.

However, changing how we think about the situation doesn't mean we have to "swallow" our emotions and not let them be seen. Not processing, or "swallowing," emotions doesn't make them go away. It simply locks them somewhere where a person cannot experience them at the moment. Instead of magically vanishing, it makes those negative experiences stack one on top of another creating negative patterns that impact one's entire life—worry, self-doubt, lack of confidence, frustration about the external world, and many more.

Suppressing emotions in any way is like cheating. A shortcut to feeling good and finding inner peace, but only for a brief moment. Once the effect wears off, we are still faced with the same unresolved problems and emotions that we try to escape from. Stimulants, bad habits and various substances people use to address their emotional states are all band-aids. Real problems surface when we take these band-aids off and remove all kinds of stimulants from our lives.

Emotional resilience is about *controlling* the responses we have to stressful situations. Everyone feels fear, anxiety, and restlessness, but what differs is that those who can emotionally regulate can control their thought process and do not allow their emotional state to drive their decision making and actions. As much as it is painful, the only path forward is the path through—regulating our emotional state by understanding and taking ownership of the response. When we make peace with ourselves in such a way we build emotional resilience, which helps us navigate future challenges and focus on what we want to do in life.

REFRAMING IN THE FACE OF PAIN: HELL WEEK OF BUD/S TRAINING

Hell Week is the U.S. Military's hardest physical and mental challenge. It is designed to take the body and mind of aspiring Navy SEALs to the absolute limit. This six-day period of Basic Underwater Demolition/SEAL Training (or BUD/S) sees over half of the trainees quitting, which is more than in the remaining seventeen months combined.[11]

By some accounts, throughout this grueling challenge trainees run more than 200 miles (320km) and do other forms of physical exercise for up to 20 hours per day. They get only 4–5 hours of sleep over the entire Hell Week and have to put up with severe exhaustion and sleep deprivation. All with one purpose: to open perspective and discover that the physical body is capable of more than people think. *If I can push my limits so far, what else can I do?*

Most of those who make it through this week go on to become Navy SEALs. But these people don't rely solely on grit or willpower to succeed. Those are finite resources and as fatigue starts to take over, the attention turns more towards physical pain, doubts, and concerns. A lot of people show up fit and determined to make it through, but still Hell Week slices through more than half of very driven candidates, because extreme fatigue caused by physical exhaustion and sleep deprivation reduces your ability to think critically and push yourself. The human body is capable of withstanding tremendous amounts of pressure, much more than we would expect of it on a regular day. It's the mind that will quit halfway through the challenge to preserve itself so to go through something that is seemingly impossible, one needs to learn to control the emotional state.

Individuals who are able to change their perspective in the face of pain or fear and not let them affect the mind will succeed at expanding its capacity. Those who are able to separate the situation from thoughts and emotions are the ones who can reach deep within and focus on the purpose when the internal voice screams "pain, sleep, cold,

---

1   *Based on the account of Erik Bertrand Larssen about Navy SEAL Training in his book "Hell Week: Seven Days to Be Your Best Self"*

hunger." For example, reframing pain as a destination and not an obstacle, changing focus to how adversity makes one stronger. Or taking the smallest action possible and completing it, using a mini-victory to generate willpower to keep going.

Such thought processes are the cornerstones of emotional regulation. The more we practice (as athletes or potential Navy SEALs) the more we will be able to focus and remain calm under immense pressure.

EXERCISE: FOUR STEPS TO EMOTIONAL FITNESS

Have you ever wondered what it would feel like to live without fear? Without doubting yourself? To have unshakable confidence, feel unstoppable and able to conquer your most aspiring dreams? Think of all the great things we could achieve if we knew we couldn't fail or at least had the guts to try. We could walk up to what could be our future spouse and strike up a friendly conversation. Or start that charity project we have always dreamed of to support animal conservation. Or even take a gap year to travel the world and let the road be our guide.

But (and there is always a but)…what if he/she rejects me? What if nobody will support me and it won't work? How will I finance the whole trip? There is always fear and emotional baggage that keeps us from achieving our most desired ambitions. Baggage is nothing more than negative emotions that prevent us from looking at the bright side and being more motivated than discouraged.

Chasing a dream is a roller coaster: it involves going through ups (excitement) and downs (feeling fearful). **However, if we treat those low moments of life the same way we would treat a physical injury, it would be much easier to navigate them.** We could use that experience as learning points for the future and not be weakened by it. There's a process to healing a physical wound—we can use this same process to heal an emotional one and become more resilient as a result.

Step 1: Establish Where the Wound Is

Being emotionally fit means not letting emotions power our life. Without finding what triggers us to feel a certain way, we won't be able to get those feelings under control.

While it might be tempting to blame external factors (competition, government, bad weather) for how they make us feel, it will not change the situation. The reality is that if we want our life to change, we have to change, no one else can do it for us. The response to a situation is generated in *our* mind and because of actions WE took and decisions WE made throughout our life, bringing us where we are. We affect our life every day by every decision we make. Our mindset is a muscle that can generate confidence and if we don't take steps to strengthen it, we will face doubts instead.

As a first step, observe your thoughts on a consistent basis and write them down. Try to find situations where you feel powerless, hopeless, or discouraged. What goes through your mind? Which emotions do these situations cause? What behaviors followed? Reflect on the past to see how you overcame emotions and recognize what helped you to do so.

Often, this step alone can bring confidence, as sometimes just labeling emotions in such a way helps us to realize that there isn't much to fear. However, emotional resilience is about learning to "roll with the punches."

Step 2: Open the Wound

Once we recognize which situations make us feel vulnerable and why, it's time to "let the devils out." Allow yourself to be vulnerable, embrace the feeling (and potential emotional pain) that a stressful situation causes and live it through to get to know it. Imagine the worst possible outcome and be honest with every detail about how you feel. If you can recall a specific stressful situation in the past—use that as a case study.

If you want to learn what are your greatest fears, follow your trail of failures. All the way to childhood, if needed.

Let your emotions guide you but do it in a productive way without seeking refuge in substances. The whole point of this exercise is to become emotionally stronger. When we "swallow" emotions we generate more fear and don't allow ourselves to adapt.

The best way to approach emotional strength is to give yourself plenty of alone time and use a diary to record everything you feel (it will be needed in step #3). A diary is by far the best listener—you can be sure it will not tell anyone and will remember everything.

You can ask yourself questions below to help you understand the emotion better:

- How did the experience make me feel?
- Am I trying to cover it up? If so, what story am I telling myself?

When we go through hardships, we discover what we are made of. We push the boundaries of what we think is possible—both physically and emotionally—and reassure ourselves that we'll be able to handle whatever comes up in life. Just one step outside the comfort zone at a time and at some point, that comfort zone will grow to what earlier felt impossible.

Step 3: Clean the Wound

So, now we know which situations cause stress, anxiety, and other negative emotions (step #1). We have felt miserable to the full extent while reliving the whole experience (step #2). Now what?

It is time to reflect and process everything—i.e., find the root cause. It is necessary to uncover the root in order to recover from experience and potential trauma, much like you would take the time off to recover from the season. As they say, breakthroughs in life happen in the moments of breakdown. Only when we have truly experienced the pain are we able to commit to a decision to put it behind us. This is where a diary becomes very useful. After "brain dumping" our thoughts and feelings on paper, it's time to review that material, find patterns and underlying problems.

The process of finding the underlying reason for the lack of confidence is simple, but very uncomfortable. We need to ask ourselves the question *why* as many times as needed until we figure out what core belief triggers the chain reaction. It is uncomfortable, because it requires us to face our deepest fears, be honest with ourselves and challenge underlying beliefs. What really triggers race day anxiety? Or causes stress before speaking in public? Or hesitation before approaching a person of the opposite sex? Why does confidence evaporate when it's time to act?

To illustrate this, I will share an example from my own experience. In my first triathlon, I crashed halfway through the bike leg and had to withdraw. To make matters worse, that crash happened just 2 weeks before my main race of the year—Half Ironman—which I trained very hard for. Luckily, after the crash everything was good physically, but I knew I had to pull my emotions together to get back on the starting line.

Here's what I asked myself:

- **Why do I feel nervous about the race?** Because I'm afraid I will crash on the bike and not finish.

- **Fair enough, why do I think I will crash?** Because something might happen that will impact me.

- **Why do I think that something might come up?** Because I'm not confident in my bike handling skills. And a lot can happen over the course of a 90-kilometer bike leg. Rain, sharp descents, potholes, etc.

- **Something always comes up during training. Why do I think I won't handle it this time?** Because there's more pressure to perform during the race and I might get reckless in the face of stress.

- **Why does the pressure bother me?** Because I'm afraid my result won't match my expectations.

There it is—expectations. I am a very competitive person and the fact that I might not produce my best performance was very hard for me to acknowledge. However, I figured that only by letting go of my expectations would I be able to put these concerns to rest. Yes, I will have to slow down on the descents and be very careful. Yes, it will slow down my overall time. But sometimes you have to slow down to eventually speed up. There were two more disciplines where I could push myself harder, and that's exactly what happened.

Step 4: Seal the Wound

Now onto the exciting part. We finally untangled our emotional response process and made peace with our past (hopefully) through reviewing our core beliefs. All of that should already set a person up for being more emotionally resilient. However, to bulletproof that state and make the leap to high emotional fitness, there's one step left, to make sure this subconscious destructive thought pattern never repeats itself.

We can do it by controlling what we place our focus on and the language we use in self-talk. In particular, by working on developing good habits and putting mechanisms in place to cultivate uplifting emotions which will squeeze out fear, doubts and complaints.

Here are some ideas:

- Create personal positive mantras and put your whole energy into repeating them.
- Visualize what success is, how it feels, and replicate the respective state.
- Use power language. Instead of telling yourself, '*I'm stressed*,' say, '*I'm excited*.' Or instead of thinking, '*I'm not ready for this*,' think, '*I can do it*.' Instead of thinking, '*I doubt*,' think, '*I'm confident*.'

All in all, do anything that will focus on taking control of the situation, changing the mental state and staying strong instead of complaining or looking for excuses. Do it early while any doubt that creeps in is still small.

Remember, this last step will only be effective if the pre-work (steps #1 to #3) has been done and we are at peace with our emotions. Otherwise, these positive affirmations will not generate enough passion to really change our life and develop the resilience we are looking for.

THE "FLOW" STATE

When we think of what makes us experience joy and excitement, it is usually a specific activity or a tangible result that springs to mind first. Whether that be finishing the marathon for the first time; traveling to a new destination; summiting a mountain; competing in an adventure race; going on a honeymoon or a date with someone special; Or even something as simple as running without pain or waking up after a restful sleep.

If our mind is somewhere else, these moments will not mean a thing and will just pass by. However, in parallel, traveling when you have to work is stressful. A date when you are not interested in a person will not go well. Waking up only to scroll through social media kills the excitement for the day, and focusing on expectations for the future makes happiness depend on a certain result (personal record, place in a race, etc.).

Tangible things are not what make us happy—not a personal record, not the amount of likes on social media, not wealth and even not the things we own. **Joy, excitement and happiness come from living, not the desire to achieve something.** It is a collection of moments where we are ecstatic and jubilant that make us feel alive and fulfilled. Moments when we are completely present and fully immersed in the activity. Very often, the best moments occur when we're pushed to our limits in an effort to accomplish something difficult, substantial, and worthwhile.

If you ask an athlete to recall one of the recent great performances, he or she would probably say it was the day when everything clicked and fell into place. One might hear, "It was simply my day. I felt on top of the world, almost invincible." They probably felt calmness, confidence in their own abilities, fluidity in movements, and awareness of what was going around. Despite being physically hard, an athlete might not want the activity to stop, because it's going so well. Imagine a tennis player who is attentive to every strike of the racket and certain where the ball goes. A swimmer who feels the pressure of the water on every stroke propelling him forward. Or even a runner who is out on the trail aware of how his foot strike breaks the sound of nature. It's almost like a deep meditative state.

If you ever find yourself completely absorbed in an activity, when it feels like it is your day and you couldn't fail, you have experienced the flow state. A feeling of complete involvement in what you're doing and absolute certainty about yourself, as if you're living at the peak of your potential. For an athlete, it can mean that a hard training session feels as if it requires less effort. Or be found in a race during which he or she feels particularly strong.

> *"Flow is the state in which people are so involved in an activity that nothing else seems to matter; the experience itself is so enjoyable that people will do it even at great cost, for the sheer sake of doing it."*
>
> — MIHALY CSIKSZENTMIHALYI

Flow is an elusive state that many stumble upon by accident. A working mother who discovered that Zumba class makes her feel energized. A workaholic who went on a hiking trip and found beauty and stillness in nature. A couple who spent their honeymoon in a surf camp and got captivated by the lifestyle. Because that state is so elusive, it's very easy to lose touch with it, turn it into a routine and let it slip if you don't know what to look for.

Often, competitive athletes who return after a long break rediscover their passion for the sport and start to experience flow more profoundly. Since they have no expectation for their fitness, they usually don't obsess with performance, data or making every session as productive as possible. They return because they miss the activity itself. In a similar way, once we focus on the process and not the outcome, magic starts to happen. We start to feel present, connect with the body, appreciate nature without music, and even engage in deep conversations.

Happiness, joy and fulfillment have a direct impact on how resilient we are. There is a limit to how much we can push ourselves against our own will, but if we learn to find joy in the process, then that resource becomes essentially limitless. Above all, such a feeling of joy and connection with your authentic self can inspire energy, creativity, and drive you to have the best experience across all areas of life. Ironically, when we learn to let go is when we experience the best results. So, do things for personal enjoyment! Lose your expectations and immerse yourself in the process. If we run to feel admired or get fast, we will spend most of the time feeling anxious or bored. On the other hand, if we do something for how it makes us feel, the boredom and anxiousness disappear, and every moment and opportunity comes within our reach.

Flow is not a constant state of mind; we live our lives going in and out of it. But after every flow experience we return with more confidence in ourselves. And that improved self-esteem is like a mini-supercompensation that makes us mentally a little stronger.

THE FLOW STATE: USAIN BOLT'S PLAYFUL APPROACH TO DOMINATING THE SPRINTING WORLD

Widely considered the fastest man of all time, Usain Bolt has won individual gold medals in 100m and 200m in three consecutive Olympic Games: Beijing in 2008, London in 2012 and Rio in 2016. At the time of this writing (2021), nobody has come close to matching his World Record times of 9.58 for 100m and 19.19 for 200m.

However, it's not the results that brought him international fame and made him an icon of the sport. Instead, it's the effortless way in which he accomplished all his feats. At the height of 195cm he stands out from the rest of the sprinters, yet it seems as if he's gliding through the air. His movements are smooth, and it looks as if he was born with the gift. By far the most exciting thing to watch is his pre-race theatrics and celebrations afterwards. Those 10 seconds of insane intensity seems no big deal for him—just an interruption in an otherwise carefree, upbeat, and joyful day. After the finish line, while his competitors are breathing heavily, he carries on running, stopping only to strike a lightning pose.

Behind that spectacle is hard work, both physically and mentally. All of the theatrics and the upbeat mood is part of Bolt's routine; it's his flow. When the pressure is on, he uses that as a means to zone out the noise and focus fully on delivering top performance for that one brief moment. Every athlete who is in the flow, genuinely enjoys whatever he or she is doing. It's just that Usain Bolt is probably one of the most vivid examples of it.

While many athletes before and after him were able to produce impressive, record-shattering performances, few of those stories match in popularity.

If there's anything that this story teaches us, it is that the more an activity looks like a game, the more enjoyable it becomes and the better we are able to focus on it. We tend to evaluate athletes based on the physical performance they produce, but more often than not it's their mental capacity that affects success. In particular, athletes who are able to enter the flow state and focus are far more likely to stay consistent, recover from setbacks and failures quicker, and overall get better results.

THE PRESENT MOMENT

Why is it that we sign up for races and pay for the opportunity to put ourselves through hard physical exercise? Why engage in extreme activities and seek adrenaline? Or seek anything in life, really? I can imagine a keen parachute jumper would answer that when you are in the air free falling towards the ground, that's when you feel like you are truly living. A surfer might say that becoming in harmony with the wave feels like finding inner peace. Personally, I still remember the goosebumps I felt on every step as I climbed a volcano at night many years ago.

What is common between these peak experiences is that they force us to be fully immersed in the moment. To forget about the rest of the world and focus only on one specific thing, even if it hurts or scares us. The tougher the ordeal, the more focus it demands and the more excited, empowered and energized we become once we complete it. We seek these experiences, because that is when we feel like we are truly living. It doesn't have to be a physical challenge for us to feel mindful in such a way. One person might feel energized when truly connecting with someone and having a passionate conversation. Another one can get uplifted while playing a musical instrument. Even a child can get so engaged in an activity that he or she becomes ignorant to everything that happens around.

Flow is the state of mind when we are fully engaged in what we do and have no doubt about ourselves. As a result, everything seems to fall into place by itself. We are aware of the environment around us, yet don't stress about it. We feel the breath and the movement of our body parts but are not concerned about getting tired. We are in tune with our body and mind and are able to channel that energy towards something. That awareness, absolute confidence and focus on the goal, make us feel almost invincible. And one doesn't need to spend a year in a monastery or jump out of an airplane to discover that inner power.

We tend to experience flow when we enjoy what we do, and we can only do that when we are fully present. While peak experiences do trigger an overflow of emotions, it's the present moment that does so, not necessarily the activity itself. That moment is always there, and when we fully immerse ourselves in it, we can control the flow state. All we need to do is let go of expectations and become mindful about it.

A refreshing run is when we connect with body, mind, and maybe even with nature. An amazing date is when there's magic, electricity and "clicking." Having a great time with friends is about having fun, laughing, and having meaningful conversations. All of it is only possible when we don't have anything on our "mental agenda," when we fully commit and immerse ourselves in the experience. That's when time stops, and we make the most of the moment.

We all have our low moments every now and then, right? Times when we don't feel like going for that run, sticking to healthy habits, or even seeing other people. When turning on the TV, opening social media, browsing through email, or even reading some "very interesting article" seems like a much better use of our time than doing what is actually important. When we have goals and ambitions that are outside of our comfort zone, such discomfort comes as a package deal. It's not easy to do the uncomfortable because our mind always looks for the path of least resistance, but that is what gets us to the next level. So, it's very useful to learn to deal with such resistance to create meaningful change in our life.

Our energy in life does not depend on what we eat or how well we sleep. It is generated from within. Our emotional state is the power that gets us out the door when we need it. Consider waking up at 5a.m. when you have to do something you do not enjoy (go to work or clean the driveway). You'll do anything to postpone the moment, but if it's for something exciting (like traveling to an exotic place), all of a sudden you find the energy.

In a passive state of mind, it's incredibly hard to get going, motivate ourselves to do anything meaningful and put the effort in. Instead, we feel apathetic, sluggish, and more eager to seek distractions. In a powerful state, however, we feel like a million dollars, energized and eager to take action on our goals.

"If you want to make it big, you've got to push yourself beyond your limits. You've got to pump yourself up and get yourself into a hyper mental state. And you have to do this yourself. Nobody can do this for you."

— TONY ROBBINS

Being able to change your emotional state at will is what sets resilient athletes apart from the rest. This ability to focus and self-regulate allows them not only to control the flow, but also helps them to perform at the highest levels.

THE WINNER'S MINDSET

Very often people unintentionally add a lot of pressure into their life by putting happiness on hold until they achieve their goals. *When I am this strong, then... When I complete this race, then... When I will earn enough money, then...* It's great to have aspirations in life, however waiting for something to happen to feel fulfilled is not what winners do. Such a mentality doesn't allow a person to feel good about oneself and assumes that he or she has already accepted defeat. They believe they are not strong enough, not fast enough, not successful enough, or not happy enough. Moreover, excitement about achievements lasts for some time, but eventually fades, and when that person starts to set new goals, he or she will once again feel incomplete.

The secret to winning—in a race or in life—is that we have to win in our heads first. To conquer our own doubts and insecurities. To get in a state of absolute certainty where defeat is not an option. Think for a moment of the champions we select to be our role models: they don't wait for something to happen and don't even entertain the thought that they might not be enough. Instead, they say, '*This is where I am and that's what I need to work on next.*'

They approach life with courage instead of starting at a disadvantage. Real winners have unshakable confidence about their abilities, which helps them do whatever it takes to win.

The reality is that we never arrive. It's an ongoing journey and none of us knows our true limits. By attaching ourselves to a certain label (i.e., not good enough) or measuring our self-esteem with artificial standards, we plant a seed of destruction in ourselves and, essentially, limit our own potential. We are much stronger than we think and can achieve much more than what we set our eyes on. Instead of meeting other standards, define your own and adopt a mentality of '*I am what I am now.*' Accept your strengths and weaknesses, create an action plan to achieve your goals and work on it. When we are at our best, others will rise to meet us.

We are not defined by our past or any label. **We choose our own identity and therefore how we grow further.** Olympic athletes make it to the top for one reason. They learned to crush their doubts and enter that powerful emotional state that makes them feel like winners. They say how we do anything is how we do everything. So, to become the best version of yourself, approach any task as you would approach the Olympic final, in the peak state and ready to deliver your absolute best.

We all have our own version of the Olympics, so let's look at the steps to create that winning mindset.

PHYSIOLOGY

Our mind and body are connected through neural pathways that control our everyday functions, from breathing and digestion to thinking and movement. That means our emotional state and the physical body are interconnected. Too much mental stress, for example, can weaken the body's immune system and make a person more susceptible to various illnesses. On the other hand, an intense training schedule can drain not only physical, but also emotional reserves and impact the mood. That can be clearly visible in our body language as well. When we slump over, keep our head down, and neglect our body, we are more likely to feel sluggish, apathetic, low on energy or otherwise negative. On the other hand, when we stand up straight with our chest out, we are far more likely to feel proud and alert.

When we feel passive or insecure, it is hard to make a change in life or put a substantial effort into chasing our dreams. However, when we feel like a million dollars, we are at the top of our game and ready to conquer the world. We have the power to change our state in an instant. That mind-body connection works both ways, which is why changing our emotional state from passive to energetic starts by changing our physiology.

The most effective way to change an emotional pattern is to do something active. It doesn't have to be a proper workout, just a few push-ups, squats, jumping jacks or even a dance break will be enough to elevate the heart rate, get blood pumping, and make you feel energized.

Another way to change physiology is to alter the breathing pattern. In particular, doing belly breathing and focusing on taking deep breaths helps to get more oxygen in. More oxygen means more energy and when we are energized, we are less likely to fall into a passive state of mind.

The third and most challenging tactic to make a change in the emotional state is to shock the body for a brief moment. Intense stress causes the release of multiple hormones (including adrenaline), but if it's kept short, it helps to energize the body. Cold exposure is a great example of that—just one minute in a cold shower can radically change your emotional state.

STRATEGY: CREATE A POWER MOVE

If you watch closely, you notice athletes doing certain movements before or after the race. They are hitting their chest, lifting their arms in the sky, making certain signs or gestures. Many are just repeating the same warmup routine over and over again. With these, sometimes strange, movements athletes are using the power of anchors to enter the flow and reach deep into their desired mental state. That of absolute confidence in which they feel unbreakable and able to deliver peak performance.

An anchor is a certain trigger to a desired internal response which is typically created during a Peak Experience. The idea behind the process is to save an empowered emotional state (flow) and everything connected to it (feelings, thoughts, sounds, etc.) and associate it with a certain movement. Once that is done and practiced enough, that powerful state can be accessed at any point of type by repeating the movement.

Imagine you went out for a run and the weather deteriorated. You planned to have a solid workout, but instead there's rain and wind. Frustrated about the fact that the workout is not going as it should, you jump and shake yourself up, saying, '*There's no stopping me,*' and start running hard. After finishing the run, you realized that the conditions and the adrenaline from the emotional state pushed you to run close to your best time for a 5K. So next time, in order to get into that same emotional state, you jump and shake yourself up again as if there's that same obstacle that requires you to power through. The same goes with music: if you were in a great mood and a certain song was playing, chances are the next time you hear it you will recall that good feeling as well.

Coaches use the power of anchors to instill a certain state, behavior or thought pattern to an athlete. You can do that to yourself as well by creating your power move.

Think of an activity that makes you feel energized and excited. Recall a peak experience or imagine yourself winning a competition you have trained hard for. You're overflowing with joy and emotion; what pose or a move do you feel like making? Fist in the air? Flexing a muscle? Imitating breaking through something? If it's music that gets you going, how do you move when your top song is playing?

Once you have an idea of a signature move, it's all about practice. The more energy you can bring to the move, the better you'll get at entering the flow. When you are in an empowered state or in a great mood, practice it to remember it. When you are in a passive state, use the move to energize yourself and recall the emotions you had when you felt on top of the world.

LANGUAGE

We speak to ourselves all the time—internally or out loud. And while we might not notice it directly, the way we do it translates into how we operate and, essentially, perform. When we ask questions like, '*Why do bad things always happen to me?*' We are more likely to feel unenthusiastic and powerless, as opposed to if we were to ask, '*What can I do to better my situation?*' The more negative self-talk we engage in, even if we mean it as a joke, the more doubt we will have about ourselves.

That self-doubt starts with the kind of language we use. Words we attach to our experience become our experience, because they determine what emotions we feel (remember, actions impact thoughts and thoughts impact emotions). That means we have the power to affect our experience by lowering the intensity of negative emotions or multiplying the effects of positive ones. So, choose the language you use to speak to yourself carefully. Break the pattern of negative thinking and always try to consider what emotions your language promotes. Instead of thinking, '*I could never do that, I guess I'm not meant for this,*' a better way to frame it is, '*I'm learning, I believe I can, I'll figure it out.*' Doing so requires effort, but with resistance comes growth.

Negative language that people use is an indicator that there is a strong discontent with their current situation, especially when swearing or cursing is involved. In other words, there is a strong desire for change that is expressed through words that carry strong emotions. That desire can serve as jet fuel for personal transformation, but only if it is used for exactly that purpose: to push through obstacles, motivate yourself to grow and move forward in life. Without action that internal desire will go to waste and only create more resentment and a feeling of powerlessness. For example, instead of thinking, '*Why is it always me who catches a cold? Now I cannot train for a week,*' think, '*I was given an opportunity to slow down, review what is not working and build myself even stronger.*'

How extraordinary your life could be if you had a superpower to diffuse negative emotions and intensify positive ones? Developing that ability starts with noticing the negative words we use on a consistent basis and changing them. For example, if you are feeling anxious or stressed in the lead up to a race, frame it as excited to race instead. Nervousness triggers the release of the hormone adrenaline which in small quantities actually improves athletic performance by activating the "fight or flight" response that prepares the body for strenuous activity. So, being excited means accepting the fact that race nerves are a normal part of delivering your best performance and at the same time, not letting the fear of not meeting expectations take over.

STRATEGY: CREATE A PERSONAL MANTRA

When we learn to control it, our mental state is not defined by external things. Whatever we think or how we perceive external events is always inside our minds. That view should never be pushed on us. Which is why the main opponent for an athlete is always within—it is the fears, doubts and insecurities that circle around in the head. If an athlete is not mentally resilient, then all the negatives will only get amplified.

Beliefs we have about ourselves have the power to build us up or to tear us down. Human beings have the awesome ability to take any experience of their lives and create beliefs that either paralyze them or empower them to take action. Since beliefs are learned, they can also be changed, especially if that improves the quality of life. And one way to shatter a belief that is no longer serving you is through language.

The word mantra comes from Sanskrit and has multiple meanings: praise, hymn, sacred message or text, song, charm, or incantation. At its core, a mantra is a sound or a phrase through which we mindfully focus our thoughts. While it is frequently used in meditation to quiet the noise, anyone can benefit from one. A mantra can help to focus thoughts on triggering a desired emotional state, especially when you create one that is meaningful to you.

To be powerful, a personal mantra needs to be spoken out loud again and again with absolute certainty. When under pressure or in times of doubt it helps to distance yourself from the cause and focus on entering an empowered state: flow. When you do it with passion, you start to believe what you're saying and become certain of it. You engage your nervous system with the full force of your focus, emotion, and body, which helps you enter into flow.

Think about the situations that make you feel stressed or in which you feel powerless. Decide what you want to be or feel instead and create a personal mantra to condition yourself to become that person. Here are some of the examples you can use:

- I am vibrant and full of energy
- I am in control of my life
- I am more powerful than my pain
- My fears do not control me
- I am becoming the best version of myself
- I am unstoppable

STORY

There is an area of our brain called the Reticular Activating System (RAS) that is responsible for filtering out unnecessary information, so that the important stuff can get through. It's the reason why we can spot a familiar person in a crowd of people or suddenly wherever we go we start hearing a song that we recently listened to on the radio and liked. The RAS, essentially, takes what we pay attention to and creates a filter for it. It then scans the environment and presents only the data that is important to us. Without us noticing, of course.

In the same way, RAS seeks information that validates our beliefs. It helps us recognize more of what we focus on and find reasons for why it's true. If you think you're a bad dancer, you probably will be. If you think you are good at cooking, you most likely are. When we doubt ourselves, life will prove it and when we believe in ourselves, we'll find success even in times of adversity.

"Whether you think you can, or you think you can't—you're right."

— HENRY FORD

As a result, whatever we consistently tell ourselves becomes our story which, over the course of many repetitions, we start to believe. A person who doesn't feel confident or worthy will tell him or herself that something is risky, today is not the day, he or she is not yet ready, the weather is bad, the economy is weak. He or she will look for every opportunity to complain, feel weak or give up and will definitely find evidence for such doubts. Hardships make us stronger only if we tell ourselves the right story—that we are resilient and are strong enough to make it through.

In life, we get whatever we focus on. If we focus on problems, we get more problems. If we focus on excellence, we become better. However, when we change what we consistently put our attention to, we can rewrite our story. Our brain will always look for the evidence to support whatever we decide to focus on. So, trade expectations for appreciation—be grateful for the experiences you have as well as the downturns because they make you who you are. Training your Reticular Activating System in such a way helps to condition the brain and tell it what's important to you, so that it can seek such experiences out.

STRATEGY: VISUALIZATION

Feeling the inner fire burning and being willing to put the effort in to achieve something often comes down to perspective. When we dare to visualize the outcome we want, we create an emotional connection with it, and it has a higher chance of materializing. Visualization (or mental rehearsal) is a very powerful tool that athletes and coaches use to improve self-confidence, motivation and create an intent behind a race or a training session.

It's a form of mindfulness meditation that aims to create a mental image of what a person wants to happen or feel. Our brain cannot really distinguish between what is real and what is vividly imagined, which is why it's important to make the experience as real as possible. We are quite literally deceiving the mind and making it believe that what we are mentally rehearsing is real. So, it's not about simply kicking back on a couch, closing your eyes and daydreaming about gold medals. Consider it a mental workout that will have a lasting effect.

Such mental imagery is an opportunity to reduce the anxiety and stress an athlete might experience when facing an uncertain situation. A competitor will run faster than expected. The weather will suddenly change. There might not be enough time to do the usual warmup. To win at something in life we first need to overcome the doubt and win in our mind. And no win comes without adversity.

Find a quiet spot and take a moment to think about and really focus on the event or competition you are preparing for. Start with the easy and less stressful part and build from there. How does your morning look? What do you do upon waking up? What will you eat? Continue with the warmup routine and then the race itself. Try to imagine your best result, be it winning or achieving a personal record. What does it take to achieve? What struggles might you come across? The next time try imagining things not going the way they should; how would you deal with it? Imagine that.

Make the mental image in your head as vivid as possible and try to "replicate" emotions, feelings, environment, sounds, anything you can think of. This emotional connection will send a message to the brain that you are worth it and the willpower and motivation will grow. Mental preparation is much like practicing a skill: the more you imagine a certain activity, the better you get at regulating the emotions associated with it. So, do it as often as possible.

Here are some tips for effective visualization:

- **Relax and clear your mind.** Visualizing what you desire is hard when your mind jumps from one thought to another

- **Use different perspectives.** Do not just visualize with your own eyes. Become a spectator and witness as it unfolds from the stands or how it would look like on television. How does your coach standing on the sideline see it?

- **Make the experience real.** Prepare for everything: what you want it to be, what you don't want it to be and what it could be. How would you change a flat tire or what would you do if you tripped and fell?

- **Engage all your senses.** The more details and sensations you can add to the visualization, the more authentic the experience becomes and the more the brain is willing to buy-in. What is the smell on race morning? How does the wind feel on your face? How cold is the water?

EXERCISE: EFFECTIVE ROLE MODELING

Looking up to someone can be a very powerful motivational trick for any situation in life, but only if done the right way. Unfortunately, what sometimes happens is that people put their role models on a virtual pedestal or even consider them "demigods," which creates a big gap between them and leads to a disempowered state. Looking at elite athletes and thinking I am not that fast, or I cannot handle such training loads is just one example of it.

More often than not, people are drawn to characters and personalities, not necessarily results. So, instead of comparing yourself to your role models (which only amplifies the lack of confidence or the feeling of anxiety), ask instead What would my role model do? Or how would my role model handle this situation? This simple change in perspective will turn the mindset from being a victim to being in control.

The most effective way to use a role model is to make yourself one. Craft the identity you desire and use your future self as a role model for the behavior and results you wish to achieve. What would you do in that empowered state? What actions, habits and thinking patterns got you to succeed? It's easy to discount someone else who has different life and interests, but you cannot deny your own life, dreams, and ambitions.

The goal of this exercise is to find your pattern for flow and create an identity around it to help you access that empowered state at will.

CREATE YOUR UNIQUE IDENTITY

First of all, remember the occasion when you felt like a winner—on top of the world with nothing holding you back. The moment when you experienced the purest joy. It might be a result of actually winning something, breaking through a limitation, or even realizing a dream. Close your eyes and relive it fully. How did you feel at the moment? What emotions were rushing through your mind? What were you thinking of and what words did you use, internally and out loud? How did you stand, sit or act in the moment? Where did you look? What song was playing in your head? What did the surroundings look like?

If you cannot recall an occasion or cannot experience it fully, imagine realizing your wildest dreams and go through the same process.

Now, try to summarize that peak experience as follows:

- **Language:** How would you describe yourself when you are at your absolute best and everything is going better than you ever imagined? Example: I am unstoppable, courageous, powerful, fearless, passionate.

- **Story:** What do you need to say to put yourself in that empowered state? Example: I will find a way, or I will make a way. I am more powerful than my pain. I am great at this; my fears do not control me.

- **Physiology:** When you are in that energized and victorious state, what power move do you feel like making? Example: fist in the air, flexing a muscle, imitating breaking a wooden board, raising arms in the air.

As a final touch, give your new empowered identity a nickname, just like performers do when they create a stage name for themselves. It can be anything but has to be meaningful to you in order to instill the desired language, story and physiology. This identity will serve as a role model that you will look up to for inspiration and strength. Who are you when you are in that Peak Emotional state? Who do you need to be to realize your dreams? Example: Doubt Crasher, Giant, Superman, Warrior, Samurai. The list is endless.

PRACTICE ENTERING THE FLOW

Once you have created your empowering identity, you need to anchor it to a movement that will help you access that feeling of flow. Every time you experience little victories, practice making your power move (the one you feel like making when you're energized) to attach emotion to it and connect to that empowered and victorious state. Besides that, practice making the same power move before any important activity: a race, a presentation at work, an important appointment or doing anything else where you might slide down to a passive state. Remember to think of the story you tell yourself and the language you use as you do it.

Over time this practice compounds and the identity you have created for yourself will help to enter the state of flow at will.

LIFE IS AN EXPERIENCE

How long do you think it would take you to swim a mile? What about 10 miles? For an advanced swimmer, that would be two days' worth of intense training. Now imagine swimming non-stop for two days while at the same time battling strong currents, venomous jellyfish and, obviously, extreme fatigue. Sounds impossible, I agree, but that's exactly what makes Diana Nyad's story so incredible. After multiple attempts, at 64 years of age she became the first woman to swim unassisted from Cuba to Florida—an epic journey of 110 miles (177 kilometers).[1] Besides the length, such a feat of endurance is considered so dangerous that most open-water experts concluded that anyone who would attempt it without a shark cage would die. *Diana didn't use one.*

During the 53 hours that the ordeal had taken, she didn't sleep and stopped only for brief moments to drink and take in some food. What makes this story even more inspiring is that before starting her training, Diana had not been swimming for thirty years. While she did make an attempt to complete the challenge at 28, she was only able to fulfil her lifelong dream after reconnecting with her fitness in her 60s. It took a total of five attempts and Diana faced adversity on every one of them: storms and currents pushing her off-course, jellyfish stings and shoulder pain, to name a few. But she never gave up and carried on because being defined by limitations was not in her plans. Every attempt was hard mentally and physically, but all that experience only made her more resilient.

---

1   Based on Diana Nyad's account of the experience in her book "Find a Way: The Inspiring Story of One Woman's Pursuit of a Lifelong Dream."

Overcoming adversity is never easy. It relies that we push through discomfort in an attempt to discover our limitations and break through them, which, let's be honest, few people actually enjoy. **But that's where the secret to growth lies: in that very thing that seems so intimidating and humbles our spirits when it's time to act.** Once we get past the initial desire to curl under a blanket with our favorite sitcom in the background and let our flow state do its magic, we start to benefit from the discomfort. We stretch ourselves, learn, adapt, and change.

The more discomfort we overcome in such a way, the more opportunity we get to practice the skill of resilience and make life more exciting, interesting, and engaging in the process. It's up to us to create those profound experience, to change situations we don't like and make a conscious effort to not repeat any of the mistakes we make.

"At the apex of the pain, that's where success is."

— ELIUD KIPCHOGE

It takes time to build a mindset to consistently break through the limitations and habits that are associated with it. But the best part is that once in place, it spreads to every area of life; if we can master discomfort, we can master just about anything. Building resilience is a slow process and, just like training, requires dedication and consistency. You do not always see progress from week to week or month to month, but that doesn't mean it's not there. Often, it is only when reflecting over a longer timespan that we can see how far we have come and what amount of pressure we can handle.

Adventures that require a certain degree of physical fitness are a great mechanism for breaking through limitations. As we push through physical discomfort, we do so in our mind as well. **Every activity or event that challenges us also forces us to learn and develop skills that in the future help us overcome a similar situation better.** Such micro adaptations become a series of supercompensation that bit by bit make us more well-rounded and resilient. Living an adventurous life provides an opportunity to have varied and more profound experiences that test us in multiple ways. When we get out of our way to try new things or let new things happen to us, our brain develops neural pathways that create more confidence and make it easier for us to go ahead with the experiences we desire truly in life. In other words, the bigger the challenges we attempt, the better experiences we get to have and, the more willing we are to step out of our comfort zone again.

But there is a lot more that goes into designing a profound experience that makes a meaningful change in our lives than simply packing your bag. For starters, it requires us to go back to our ambitions and ask ourselves What is it that I really want?

CASE STUDY: ADVENTURE VS. HEART ATTACK

John approached me for coaching with an interesting request—to support him in designing an active lifestyle that is sustainable. His exact ask was, "To be super fit, have a long healthy and happy life, and to teach/encourage others to follow." John has just turned 60 and was a lifeguard and ski patroller in his earlier days, he was interested in any activity, be it running, cycling, rowing, or skiing. A non-typical athlete, with an itch for adventure, a desire to better himself and no particular interest in the competitive side of sports.

I was excited to support John because his ambitions fit very well with my vision of helping people become all-around resilient athletes and fit enough to take up any life challenge. But there was an elephant in the room: 2 years earlier, John had suffered a heart attack that had shaken his confidence. In particular, one of the concerns was whether he can regain his fitness with exercise at his age.

When his cardiac rehab finished, the first thing John did was transition to a plant-based lifestyle. He was determined to make a change in his life and after organizing his nutrition, he turned to exercise and got himself a heart rate monitor. The purpose was really strong: to change the lifestyle, get in peak shape and, ultimately, become an adventure and outdoor experience guide for youth and adults. That inner fire was spot on, but we had a big gap to close, for which we needed a lot of discipline, focus, and small wins.

Together, we started off by creating a fitness regime that included a wide range of daily physical activity like rowing, cycling, rucking and, eventually, running. In a span of six months, John went from very minimal exercising to consistent 5-hour weeks—more time than many amateur and hobby-athletes twice as young spend training. It wasn't always glamorous, and the progress wasn't linear, but gradually his running improved to a point where he could complete a 10-mile run with ease. As he said himself, "The training process helped me understand my body better and made me feel that I can overcome limitations and still do all of the exciting things I intended to." More importantly, as he got fitter, his physician also gradually reduced the blood pressure medication he was on.

In general, peaking in one's 60s is somewhat of a rarity, but some, John included, do manage to hold on to or even improve their fitness as a result of (or for the purpose of) leading an adventurous life. And that's a good indicator of a resilient athlete. John had a lot of limitations that had the power to put down any spark of inspiration or passion. The emotional burden of a recent heart attack, medication that affected performance, lack of experience with training programming, doubts, and limiting beliefs related to his age.

However, what he lacked in physical resilience, he compensated with the strength of his character. An easy solution for him would be to reduce stress, don't overload the body too much and maybe find a calm hobby to stay entertained. Instead, he chose to take the longer route and break through every limitation with a gradual approach. Not by running hard in an attempt to get back into shape quickly, and not by going on a detox diet to lose weight quickly. John built his physical resilience by changing his lifestyle one small step at a time and gradually made it to the point where he's comfortable exercising more than he ever did, prepared to embark on even greater adventures and overall feeling his best ever self.

SET INSPIRING GOALS

Athletes who have achieved a high level of fitness are very often meticulous about every aspect of their performance. Every little detail is considered, tracked, and analyzed—the length of speed and recovery intervals, duration of each training session, strength gains, gear and its condition, timing of nutrition, and much more. Personally, I believe in such a professional approach to anything, because that dedication cannot fail to bring results. Probably because I'm so scrupulous myself and it's the legacy competitive sports left on me. What if we apply such diligence to fulfilling our dreams? Planning and setting up our experiences so that they move us closer to our vision? Develop the skills and knowledge needed to attempt more challenging endeavors that advance us further? Don't shy away from taking action? Every conscious effort starts with a goal.

They say without a goal you can't score. Without knowing what it is that you want to achieve, it's hard to figure out how to do it. Our purpose and vision of the life we want to lead serve as our North Star. Designing an active lifestyle that's not only exciting, but also sustainable and fulfilling requires that we set our goals and plan our experiences as milestones that move us closer to fulfilling that vision. Once we do that, we become excited about reaching them. After all, we desire progress, which is why we set goals in the first place. That progress has to be towards something meaningful and important to us. Otherwise, what's the point?

Moreover, when we set a series of smaller goals this way, we make the process of achieving our vision more interactive, almost like a quest. It brings us closer to the present moment and to that empowered state of flow. When we enjoy the process, making the necessary changes or sacrifices will not be that difficult. We start to wake up every morning feeling grateful and energetic, even if it means doing so earlier to squeeze a training session in. That's when we become empowered to take control of our lives and develop a mindset to do anything to fulfil our dreams.

There are two types of athletes: those who withdraw from a race if it doesn't go as expected or gets too intense and those who finish no matter what place they come in. The same goes for life. There are people who quit because they don't see quick progress and those who adjust their effort but stick till the end. To think about it, isn't it crazy to abandon a dream just because it's too ambitious?

There is a mental trick that athletes use in a race, or during a particularly hard training session, to get over a hard patch. When the pressure is high and everything hurts, they try not to think about how much distance is still left to cover. Instead, they focus on one small bit at a time—run to the next turn, swim to the next buoy, or even count the steps—and immerse themselves in the present moment. **In a similar way, breaking down a vision into smaller parts makes it less intimidating and more achievable.** Splitting the vision into many smaller and easily attainable goals creates stepping stones to that intimidating peak we are chasing. It helps to fully focus on the next immediate action and later appreciate the resilience that each smaller experience has helped to build. When I first came up with the idea to finish an Ironman, 10 hours of non-stop exercise felt very intimidating. But after completing three marathons, crashing in my first triathlon, and finishing a half Ironman race, the whole idea didn't seem that crazy anymore.

These goals can be as small as you want—nobody is there to judge. The most important thing is that a) they are on the way to (support) a bigger vision/life goal and b) you are able to complete them with ease. In fact, setting a few small goals with short timelines is a very effective way to generate momentum and break patterns that no longer serve you. That's why challenges, such as "1,000 push-ups in 30 days" or "detox weeks" are so popular. They focus on one small and easily achievable goal and attach a short timeline to it that keeps people focused. **However, this approach will only work if the goal or challenge fits with the purpose you have developed.** Otherwise, those micro habits will not stick and will not grow into a change you want to see in your life. And that is when people find themselves running in circles, jumping from one challenge to another without seeing much progress. Remember the Circle of Life? Every outcome we get originates in our mind and is driven by beliefs we have about our potential.

Having a goal is not enough, though. Every worthy one needs a plan of action. People do not climb Mount Everest by flying to Nepal and trekking up it. Reaching the summit requires a lot of planning and preparation even before boarding a plane. It helps to think of achieving goals like a mountaineering expedition. Plan your route (map out smaller milestones) in advance, consider the resources that you will need along the way, think of the people who can support you, things that can go wrong, and how you would manage them.

Be careful not to get stuck in the planning phase or get caught by the analysis paralysis—to plan something and then re-plan whatever was planned because things have changed. This lack of momentum is often what stops people from making progress in their vision. The strategy to avoid this is to conclude the planning phase with immediate action. Think about one big bold step you can take right now to make the goal possible and jump right into the action by taking it.

THE VALUE OF REINVENTION

Resilience is a capacity that is honed by consistently balancing on the tightrope that is the edge of the comfort zone. Throwing yourself out of balance by trying something new and then bringing it back to harmony with the power of emotional fitness. Diligent practice forges a superpower, and a robust growth mindset that lays the foundation for an authentic and purposeful life. Resilient athletes know that the peak they are working towards (no matter how ambitious) is not the end of their journey but rather just a milestone on the path to something even bigger. They might not know yet what it is or what to expect, but they accept such uncertainty and are open to experimentation.

> *When we consistently change the course of our life and subject ourselves to uncertainty, we enrich our life and become stronger in the process.*

In reality, the only way we can learn what we are good at, what we are meant to do, and even what we want to do, is through experience. The more diverse, the better. Whenever we focus on that goal race or put our heart and soul into the training process, we should remember that there's always a bigger world out there. Excitement about a personal record or any other achievement lasts for a while, but eventually fades away. And when it does, it's time to look for a different challenge, not necessarily one that is physically harder, but one that will help us grow further.

For any athlete, reaching peak physical fitness is high on the lifetime goals list. But that peak can be so much more than beating a personal best or dropping below 10 percent body fat. **When we overfocus on one specific thing or get too comfortable, we start to stagnate and eventually decline.** A resilient athlete is a well-rounded one and is capable of using his fitness not only to perform well in a race, but also in life to have more profound and valuable experiences. Which is why trying as many things as possible and having diverse experiences ensures that we grow not only in performance, but also in perspective.

Reinventing means transforming yourself from the inside out with a goal to keep growing and consistently find the answer to the question, "What do I want to become next?" Sometimes that means switching disciplines (like moving from a 5K to a marathon), but often it means switching sports altogether. While it can be scary to start something new, the only way to grow is to evolve past experiences so that they are not holding us back. The quest for resilience, therefore, should make a person struggle and teach them something new about him or herself, not only in a physical sense. That challenge is what makes us immerse ourselves in the moment and is often the best part of the whole journey.

So, how to find ways to reinvent yourself? Well, if you are struggling with this question, a great place to start is to list down all the things you either don't like to do or are uncomfortable doing, and then to do them. Especially those things that you know are good for you. Yes, often that would mean doing something that is not fun, like waking up before dawn to exercise or batch prepare food for the week. But don't get discouraged and expect to instantly master the behavior you wish to cultivate. Real change doesn't happen like that. Instead, it unfolds bit by bit, one small step outside your comfort zone at a time. And when you do that consistently, you will not fail to notice your entire lifestyle gradually changing.

In our daily life, we tend to focus more on our strengths rather than weaknesses. Reinventing yourself means using the opportunity to transform your weaknesses into your strengths.

The more often you get uncomfortable, the more resilient you will become.

There are three ways to respond to a challenge—freeze and remain where you are, retreat, or push forward. So, embrace the challenge before it pushes you back in life. Sign up for something instead of aimlessly scrolling in search of the best pair of running shoes or new training gear. Turn your thinking around and develop a mindset of befriending the obstacles, for they make you who you are. Embrace the uncertainty and make it a priority to try something new—bring yourself out of balance and let your emotional fitness do the work. The best part is that you don't have to do it alone. Involve others by telling a friend, "I'm walking 6 miles this Saturday" or, "I'm running a half marathon in 6 months." Make it concrete and have someone to keep you accountable for it.

REINVENTING THROUGH LIFE: LAIRD HAMILTON'S QUEST FOR CREATIVITY IN SURFING

Laird Hamilton is what you would call an Aquaman: he is as confident in the ocean as one can be in ever-changing conditions. Best known for his big wave endeavors, he was never a fan of the competitive side of surfing and chose to take a more playful approach to sport. His lifelong quest for trying new things enabled him to shape many iterations of what surfing can be. Most prominently, such innovations as tow-in surfing, stand-up paddle boarding and hydrofoil boarding.

Motivated by how he measures up against what's possible or what he's capable of, he managed to become a professional athlete on his own terms, without the aura of competitiveness around it. As surfing was gaining popularity with various competition formats, Laird stayed true to the playful nature of surfing and connected with joy instead. He noticed that being competitive slows down innovation, because nobody wants to try new things when their career depends on delivering the best performance. Innovating, on the other hand, implies that you risk and do something that might not work out. The same happens in life: whenever the competitive aspect takes over, we stop innovating. We focus on performance and resist trying something new. We only stick to what we know works. Unfortunately, such competitiveness prevents us from taking a step back, putting things into perspective and seeing what the best step would be to ensure growth. It limits our long-term progress, because even though something new is hard at the beginning, it might enable much more in the future.

Athletes are often reminiscent on the past and their glory days, previous wins, the medals, and the struggles. However, you rarely hear them talk much about the future, especially after ending their careers. Reinvention is a great way to make the transition smooth and remain in sports throughout your entire life. It helps to leave the competitiveness aside, understand that we do not need anyone's approval to be fulfilled and focus on what we truly want. To focus on what brings us joy. To be in the moment and not stuck in the past trying to prove something.

Laird Hamilton is a great example of a resilient athlete. His ongoing quest to do something he hasn't done and continuously push his limits made him an icon for reinvention and resilience. He inspired thousands of surfers and non-surfers to seek their own path and design life on their own terms. To do what they do in their own unique way. More importantly, thanks to the constant change of direction and what fitness means to him, he managed to keep himself engaged in surfing for more than 45 years. By exposing himself to different experiences and looking to try something new, he managed to find purpose in uncertainty and make peace with it.

THE POWER OF A TEAM

Having ambitions and staying true to yourself is a great way to push through limitations or overcome obstacles that inevitably come up in daily life. But let's be real, not everyone has an army-like discipline and willpower made of steel. Everyone experiences moments of weakness from time to time and struggles with the motivation to do what's right. While being a lone ranger might sound heroic and inspiring, as humans we thrive on communication and the sense of togetherness. **We need to spend time around people, interact or just have someone to share our successes and concerns with.** Ironically, we'll often work twice as hard to make someone else happy than we would ourselves (or at least to prove something).

Quite literally, external accountability means being obliged to meet certain expectations or report to someone. It can result from having relationships or agreements with others and is based on such values as respect, integrity, reliability, and trustworthiness. In other words, being accountable to others means respecting them and being true to the commitments you have made, which is totally different to being driven by your own values and ambitions. Having someone you don't want to let down is a great way to boost motivation when you're not feeling like it. Often, that is all that's needed to remain consistent. Which is why being a part of a peer group, a training squad, or simply having a training partner, is a more effective and enjoyable way to train. Especially when others play the game harder than we do.

And that's where the power of a team is—it pushes an athlete to become the best version of him or herself while also supporting when that person feels down. We don't need to struggle in an attempt to achieve everything on our own. In fact, those who have the courage to leave their ego aside will notice that the result of a team effort is always much greater than that of an individual. Creating a circle of people that will accept, support, and challenge us is very powerful, because those who we spend time with influence who we become. It makes the experiences that we have in life more substantial and worthwhile. If we want to achieve our goals, we need to be around people who can help us make it happen—we need to make them part of our team.

Sharing our goals with people we trust adds an additional level of accountability. Which is why a team is not necessarily a formal group, but rather a support system we create for ourselves. One of the reasons why working with a coach or having a mentor is so effective is that being accountable to someone who believes in you is a powerful motivator. Often, it's the people that we respect that we do not want to let down. A mentor and a coach are invested in our success, both as an athlete and a personality, and are valuable members of our support team. They want us to realize our potential and are willing to offer their time, knowledge, and experience to help us achieve that.

A meaningful journey is a shared journey. Involving others in whatever we do makes the experience more than just about ourselves. People go through similar experiences in life and are looking for like-minded people to associate themselves with. There's a high chance someone is facing the same problem and needs support. Or vice-versa, can offer it. A great way to leverage the power of external accountability is to let people follow your progress. Launch a like-minded well-being community and lead personal transformation by example. Or start a public blog and post consistently in it. Sharing your journey with others or just making it public may seem scary at first. *'Am I worth it? How will people react? What if they make fun of me?'* But those fears are just that—fears, nothing more. The purpose of stating our ambitions to others is to let people challenge and support us. To make them part of our team and make the experiences we have in life more enjoyable and meaningful.

KEEP IT FUN

We live in a hasty world, rushing to achieve goals, realize ambitions, or as some might say, keep up with the pace of the world. In the current age, more so than ever. Study, work, hopefully leave time for family, friends and training, and then repeat—five, six or even seven days a week. Stripping life down to bare necessities like this can take fun and joy away from it pretty quickly, making it serious, monotone and somewhat predictable. It's very easy to get stuck in this and not have time or interest to enjoy the little things. Constantly worry about what happens in the world. Be afraid of tripping down, making mistakes or looking silly.

The word resilience is often thrown around as an ambiguous buzzword to help cope with the situation when life is no longer fun. As a result, its definition was unconsciously extended to the act of persevering without complaint or even questioning. Suck it up. Push through the discomfort. Work hard now, rest later. However, more pressure, expectation to deliver and doing what's uncomfortable on a consistent basis, can sometimes become a little too much to bear. And gradually, it can become harder and harder to motivate yourself to carry on. Just like with physical overtraining, a person experiencing burnout might feel that his or her capacity to push through is decreasing. **But being resilient doesn't always mean pushing yourself to do something against your will.**

Athletes cannot stay in their peak shape throughout the entire season because it pushes the body and mind into overdrive. Be it in sports or not, people can get tired both physically and emotionally. Especially when they keep going indefinitely without giving themselves ample time to recover. Sometimes it can feel that the best thing to do is to curl up under a blanket, turn on our favorite show, take a nap, and wake up when it's all over. If that's the case, a person needs downtime immediately. Just like with physical overtraining, they need to recover, sleep, eat good food, work on becoming more mindful, maybe even do a digital and emotional detox to distance him or herself from stress. Essentially, to have the courage to switch off and let the body and mind heal. The world will still be there when you decide to re-join.

Resilience is not about never being disturbed and keep on going whatever the odds. **Instead, resilient athletes have a high level of physical and emotional awareness that helps them to know when to take the foot off the pedal and prevent overtraining or burnout.** If life is already turbulent, they don't add more stress and expectation to it by taking up a new project or training hard for an event. They give themselves space to focus on processing the events and mentally "super-compensating." More often than not, the pressure in life is ongoing and does not have a fixed start and end date. However, so is the training process; besides a few planned weeks a year, we never fully stop training. Instead, when we are tired, we adjust the intensity, take a few days easy and do some additional activities to promote recovery. We do not succumb to the pressure but learn to navigate it.

A resilient person is a happy person internally. Such individuals are energetic and motivated to overcome limitations, not because that's the way to stay afloat, but because they genuinely enjoy the process of learning what they are capable of. Having fun helps to immerse yourself in the moment and enter the flow state, a very critical component in having a peak experience. And being able to transform an activity into a game that has a fun component in it is an indicator of a resilient person.

Taking things lightly is an indicator of strength—not weakness.

Allow yourself time to have some fun; it helps you to recover and process everything that happens in life. Add back the little things: appreciate and celebrate achievements or excellent performance, however big or small it is. Such celebrations serve as something to look forward to and is a great way to recover, see where you have come from, and how much you have grown. Without appreciating small achievements, it is easy to reach a certain level of success only to realize that the journey gave more fulfilment than the actual result.

What do you do after having that peak experience? At first, you close the Circle of Life: reflect, learn, and adapt before starting a new one. Then you build a lifestyle around it to make sure you introduce it into your life on a frequent basis and with that, enrich it.

SNEAK PEEK: OBSESSION OVER PERFORMANCE

Back when I was a kid, nothing seemed to hold me in any sport for long. For me it was just a fun way of spending time. Kayaking was no exception; at the beginning it was just sun, water, time with friends, swimming and laughing. One day, however, something clicked and competitive kayaking became everything I thought about and all I wanted to do in life—all day, every day. And several years later, there I was, multiple times national champion, top 20 places in European and World championships. I was eager to see where I could take myself and how far I could go. However, at some point I noticed that something was not going right. That spark and joy I felt from doing what I love started to fade away and the whole passion turned into obsession. I was putting in more effort than ever, saying no to any excuses and refusing to listen to my body. Words like "bad weather," "fatigue," or "lack of time," were not in my vocabulary.

I thought I did what all top athletes do: train hard and give your best. Yet, it felt strange. I stopped progressing, got over-trained frequently and started to suffer from illnesses and injuries more often. I rarely struggle with motivation, but that really got to me. As I was using all my energy on training, I grew more frustrated by not seeing the expected results. I wouldn't accept any jokes about my intense schedule or healthy lifestyle and in general, interacted and smiled less. I was getting frustrated when small things didn't go as planned, and overall, kayaking started to become something I had to do, not something I chose to do. I had every intention to push through it, like I always did, but I felt as though it was not' that simple.

Being very ambitious, I never allowed myself to take a long break from training. Not more than a week or two at the end of a season. But after suffering 2 illnesses in a row just before the European Championship, I finally learned that repeating the same mistake and expecting different results is crazy. I had to change something to fix it. So, as much as I didn't want to, I stopped training and focused on studying, working, and traveling instead. I did this for a full six months to rethink what I really wanted. It brought me back to life. When I was traveling, kayaking and competing was not in the picture anymore. Instead, I found passion in trying out new things, like running, surfing, swimming, and cycling. As I started to explore these new sports, I understood that it was the way of living that brought me to competitive kayaking in the first place. Working towards a goal, doing something active, having fun doing it and becoming the best version of yourself—not necessarily the records and results.

Among other things, being resilient means not letting a single thing become your entire world and wipe out the ability to see things in perspective. Obsession in life comes from trying too hard to live life in a particular way and as a competitive athlete. For a while I was stuck in this way of thinking. I always felt like I wasn't enough and am only allowed to celebrate once I win or achieve the highest ambition that I set for myself. So, more often than not, I had a bitter aftertaste from was actually a pretty good performance. Yes, having goals and ambitions is important, but it's even more important what kind of person we become along the way and where these goals will lead us, because we'll have to live with that person inside us for the rest of our life. Do I think how good my performance would have been had I gone back to kayaking? Not really, but I know that the experiences I had as a result of moving forward helped me grow and continue to make me who I am, and I wouldn't change anything about it.

EXERCISE: THE 5-STEP FORMULA FOR CREATING MEANINGFUL EXPERIENCES IN LIFE

Have you ever felt as if you are running around in circles? Making excuses and promising yourself to start exercising tomorrow? Not trying out something new because "it doesn't seem interesting?" Chasing the next finish line or adventure with a goal to run away from problems?

It is as if we are following an old program that we installed some time ago. We might have installed it with good intentions—maybe even to make a change in our life—but as our life progressed, the program became outdated. In the meantime, a new program was not installed and instead of doing the uncomfortable, we repeat the same thing over and over again, often expecting different results.

However, if we do what we have always done, we won't grow and won't adapt to bigger challenges. Growth comes from increasing the magnitude of the experiences we have, which is in our control. Changing the program that doesn't serve us is about challenging our assumptions and beliefs. A meaningful experience is one that pushes us to the edge and forces us to reflect, learn and adapt.

There are several factors that impact the profoundness of the experience and with that the effect it has on our lives. This exercise is designed to help you craft one that will trigger a shift in your life.

Step 1: Set an Inspiring Goal

Goals typically begin as random thoughts. They keep re-appearing in our heads until we recognize a pattern and turn them into wishes and desires. However, without a deadline these are just that—wishes and desires.

A good way to structure these random thoughts, make them more specific and actionable is to use the SMART goal framework. According to that every goal has to be:

- **Specific:** With a clear outcome
- **Measurable:** Progress has to be clearly visible

- **Achievable:** Realistic
- **Relevant:** Should matter to you and be in line with your purpose
- **Time-Bound:** With a deadline attached to it

Think of what you want to have or achieve if you knew you couldn't fail. Let the inspiration flow and list down all the crazy ideas that come to mind. When finished, select one or a few that resonate most with your purpose and organize them according to the framework above.

Here's a tip: Try to avoid setting restrictive goals (i.e., lose weight or quit smoking). While the motivation behind is usually strong, this strategy rarely works. Focusing on what we need to give up is not that inspiring. When we're working to get away from something, time slows down and we tend to dread the experience. However, if we are moving towards what we really want, time flies and we're more likely to find the energy to do it. So, frame the goals in a positive way and make sure the focus is on what you get to do and not on what you're giving up (i.e., learn stand-up paddling, cook three healthy meals per week yourself).

Step 2: Plan the Entire Adventure

A plan has the power to bring the goal to life. It essentially splits the entire journey into many smaller parts that are easier to focus on and execute. Having a plan ensures that every important detail is considered, which reduces the pressure and allows a person to immerse him or herself in the present moment and fully enjoy the experience.

The process of planning can seem long and tedious. However, when we plan something meaningful and inspiring, we tend to enjoy it. In such an empowered state, it is not difficult to consider small details, because they come to mind on their own.

Think about that meaningful goal you have set and create a plan for how you would attempt to complete it. Approach it as if you were designing your ultimate experience. Split it into as many little goals as needed and try to consider every detail—what has to happen for the goal to be reached, what resources would you need, who can support you, how long it will take, what specific steps you need to do.

Finally, while still in an empowered and excited mindset think of one big and bold action you can take right now to kick the entire process off and do it or schedule it right away.

Step 3: Add a Dose of Challenge

Our mind and body need to be challenged, otherwise they will stagnate. In fact, without pushing ourselves to do something uncomfortable, we will fall behind because the world around doesn't wait for us to catch up. A lot about taking physiological or emotional fitness to the next level is about levelling up in our minds first, which is where adventure comes into play.

It's in those moments when we are challenged, that we grow. So, craft a vision of adventurous life you want to lead and create a series of mini challenges that bring that vision closer to reality. Stay ahead of what might come and challenge yourself before life challenges you.

Be open and curious. Use your imagination and sprinkle adventure throughout your life by committing to trying something new, taking spontaneous trips, or saying yes to something that scares you.

Step 4: Share Your Journey

Many pro athletes agree that having a community that pushes you is one of the most effective ways to become a better athlete. Training with a group adds a bit of competitiveness to the whole training process and, in a way, makes it seem easier and fun.

Having training partners that you don't want to let down also helps you to remain focused and keep the motivation strong. You will work much harder to keep up and not fall off the pack than you would alone.

An experience that is shared carries more power, so make an effort to involve more people in your journey. Join a training squad, find a mentor, hire a coach, start a blog, or even create a movement.

Step 5: Celebrate Accomplishments

Finally, plan how you will celebrate your achievements and reward yourself. Have fun with it and make an effort to celebrate even the smallest of accomplishments—on a daily basis. Being in good spirits is a signal that your life is in a good place.

In fact, a good place to begin is to start seeing humor around you. Don't take anything thrown at you personally and look for opportunities to make jokes instead of complaining. Have some laughs, spend time with friends, add more music to your life (the kind that motivates you to sing or dance along). Don't care about what people think, and don't take life too seriously. A year later, almost all problems we face now won't matter, so we might as well find humor in them.

PART II

Lifestyle

GENERATING MOMENTUM

We tend to think of high-performance athletes as superhuman, a rare species with a lucky gene or a strategy that's out of reach for mere mortals. But if we were to ask an elite athlete what is his or her secret to extraordinary strength and a preternatural ability to suffer, the answer will, most likely disappoint us. And that is because there is no golden strategy, shortcut, or elevator to the top, be it in fitness or life in general. The secret to high-performance doesn't come down to cutting-edge training plans, world-class coaches, carefully calculated nutrition, or even top-of-the-line recovery gadgets. It is instead found in what they call the daily grind. Showing up for good and bad days. Staying consistent with healthy lifestyle habits. Becoming a little better every time in the quest to optimize every aspect of the lifestyle. And, yes, seeking out and celebrating the pain cave, that deep place of physical and emotional discomfort that most go to great lengths to avoid. Day in and day out. Pretty boring, right? Which is why so few athletes actually do it.

We have agreed that how you do anything is how you do everything, so while at the first glance, the choices we make each day look like a result of conscious decision making, in reality more often than not we are living on autopilot. Our life is full of habits: deliberate choices we made at some point in time and then stopped thinking about. We tend to cook a certain selection of meals we learned, to go to sleep at a certain hour, and exercise in a certain way. Each of the habits on its own might not sound significant but compounded over time, they can have an enormous impact on our health, performance and even the quality of life we lead.

The life of an athlete is even more repetitive. That daily grind usually comes down to several workout types that gradually make an athlete better. **But since it's so physical, poor lifestyle habits are more visible and it's easier to discover areas where more ground can be made.** For example, if our energy levels are low as a result of lack of sleep or poor nutrition practices, we won't be able to show up at our best. Which is why even a small detail, or a habit change can trigger a series of incremental shifts (the snowball effect) that leverage the lifestyle to a whole new level.

A little push in the right direction can be all that matters.

Up to this point, we have been taking steps to create a mindset around becoming more resilient, which includes creating a purpose and establishing personal standards, learning to self-regulate and enter the flow, and, of course, embracing the pain and discomfort. This part of the book will help to create a sustainable lifestyle which leverages that mindset and makes the athlete strong and healthy. The key to achieving such sustainability is in ingraining empowering behaviors and developing healthy daily habits, which requires the same level of focus and intention as we put into our physical training. It's important to view the training program as part of the broader environment and not as life's single focus. The goal is to pay attention to and balance all aspects that impact performance: sleep, nutrition, time management and other practices.

Resilient athletes invest time in building a strong foundation in all aspects of performance, not only physical training. They recognize that what they do besides sports will have a direct impact not only on their immediate fitness, but also their health in the long term. Yes, they incorporate good training practices (i.e., stretching, cross training, strength training, and form drills) to improve the effect of exercise. But besides that, they recognize the power of lifestyle and incorporate healthy behaviors (like getting quality sleep or optimizing diet) into their lives. Imagine a rocket. It requires a massive amount of energy to start moving, but once it's in orbit momentum carries it forward. Small incremental adjustments to the lifestyle is the energy we put into generating that momentum which will carry us around the orbit of high performance.

HARD WORK BEATS TALENT WHEN TALENT DOESN'T WORK HARD

Back in 1993, Swedish psychologist, K. Anders Ericsson studied world-class performers across various fields and discovered that there seems to be one distinct commonality among them: years of practice. To be precise, on average it took 10,000 hours of consistent practice for a performer to achieve the world-class level. That is an astonishing amount which translates to roughly 3 hours every day for 9 years straight. A lot of work, but not something that's unattainable. Heaps of people start organized training at around 7–10 years of age, which means they accumulate 10,000 hours by the time they reach their twenties. So, how come there aren't that many athletes whom we tend to think of as "superhuman?" Is it natural talent that allows only a selected few to squeeze out more from their bodies? Not necessarily.

It's not just those extra hours that make someone a top performer. A more important aspect is what a person does with their time and how much quality work he or she puts into the process. **Ericsson called it deliberate practice: conscious repetition of an activity with the purpose of improving performance, and that's exactly what great athletes do.** They don't just show up to pass the time, but instead proactively search for every possible area of improvement that can influence the end result. Nothing gets overlooked, not strength, endurance, speed, flexibility, range of motion, form and alignment, core strength, agility, etc. And the quest for self-improvement doesn't end with the training process. Daily schedule, recovery, nutrition and even stress management are some of the factors that add up to create a gap between a great athlete and an average one who practiced the same number of hours.

Becoming a fast, strong, resilient, and even competitive is not a quick process, yet perfectly achievable by anyone with a strong intent and a growth mindset. It is not even subject to whether a person has the "natural talent" or not. What separates top athletes is their commitment to the process over a prolonged period of time and a lifestyle that supports high performance. At its core, any success story is the same. It's rooted in practice, the daily grind of mundane things that athletes need to get right until, eventually, all of a sudden, things click into place resulting in what others will see as an overnight success. This effect manifests in every area—sport, business, or even music—because the principles are the same. The only talent that matters is the readiness to repeat something a thousand times to make it right.

"Fear not the man who has practiced a thousand kicks once, but fear the man who has practiced one kick a thousand times."

— BRUCE LEE

Improving fitness is largely a function of tolerating more workload, be it intensity, duration, or both. As the athlete increases his training efforts over time, the body adapts and improves, bit by bit allowing an athlete to attempt even more demanding sessions. In the same way, to maintain a certain level of fitness all the person needs to do is keep the overall training load more or less constant. If you don't use it, you lose it. A hobby-runner whose experience in the sport is limited to jogging a few laps around the park on a sunny day will struggle to finish a 1-hour interval session. It will probably push him or her to the edge and will require a few days of rest to physically and emotionally recover. For an experienced athlete, however, that's a regular #tracktuesday, a weekly occurrence that's usually followed by an easy run the next day.

There are many differences between people who run zero miles per week, people who run 50 miles per week and people who run 100 miles per week. And having free time is not one of them—Yuki Kawauchi and Gwen Jorgensen are probably the best examples of that. Yuki is known in the world as the "Citizen Runner" and, among other great achievements, has won the prestigious 2018 Boston marathon while working a full-time government job and training in his free time at his own expense. Gwen, on the other hand, juggled a corporate tax accountant job and intense triathlon training that qualified her for the 2012 Olympic Games in London. She went on to win the Olympic gold four years later in Rio de Janeiro after turning professional and pausing her accountant career. A lot of people have jobs, family, and life commitments, but what distinguishes high-performance athletes and allows them to sustain an intense training schedule is the lifestyle they lead.

Unless we put our entire lives on hold, complete all the tasks in our to-do list, or win a lottery, there is never a time when we can focus exclusively on training. Which is why a more effective strategy is to integrate it and build a lifestyle around physical exercise. Otherwise, we risk not doing it at all. Athletes who structure their life around exercise approach daily decisions differently. How much they sleep, what foods they eat and even how they spend their free time is geared towards becoming the best version of themselves.

Everyone can adopt that athletic lifestyle, as it largely comes down to two areas:

- **Listening to the body.** Fitness is a moving target. The body will feel different every day, depending on many factors: training process, stress, weather, etc. Recognizing the signals that it sends us instead of muting them is a very handy skill that can help athletes make intelligent decisions about when to push themselves a little more and when to back off and take it easy. Knowing what the body can handle at each point in time helps to take each training session and make it super-effective.

- **Optimizing energy.** In particular, reducing energy waste, so that we can use it for training, recovery or all-around being our best selves. Lack of sleep, a diet that's low on nutrients, poor hydration, mental pressure,- all of these and many other harmful factors or habits cause stress and require extra energy to process. That energy can be used more effectively, therefore, athletes go to great lengths to fine-tune their schedule and make their lifestyle less taxing.

Not everyone looks at sports and wellness in such a way because it's much harder to proactively look for ways to improve oneself than to just show up and do the usual. Starting a healthy initiative is easy and the New Year's resolution movement is evidence for that. However, ingraining those practices into the lifestyle and maintaining them over a longer period of time is laborious as it challenges our existing patterns and habits. One day we want to change the world and have all these grand plans to learn surfing, backpack across Southeast Asia, kayak among the Fjords or walk the Camino de Santiago. Next thing we know, it's Thursday night and we are watching an episode of a TV series with an Oreo in one hand and flipping through social media with another. What happened? Why is it so hard to move from, "Sounds like a great idea" to, "I can't believe I'm actually doing it?"

THE MAGIC OF 1%

Subconsciously, our mind doesn't like change; anything new is always scary. This ancient pattern of thinking dates back to prehistoric times, when leaving the cave would mean accepting the risk of being eaten by a lion or any other predator. Back then, the human brain had essentially one goal, to keep us safe. While over time we evolved and developed other areas that made it possible to feel emotions (limbic system) and plan ahead (neocortex), the oldest part of the brain, the reptilian brain,[1] still affects our daily life. In fact, it is located

---

1   Based on the Triune Brain theory introduced in the 1960s by the American physician and neuroscientist Paul D. MacLean.

closest to the stem, which in the moment of danger makes our actions happen before we even think about them.

If we follow our instincts, we are programmed to hide from dangers, to remain in the comfort of the cave and be safe. That's why instead of adopting new and healthy practices, we prefer to stick with the less-than-optimal lifestyle choices that are so familiar: staying up late and getting less sleep than the body needs, eating late at night or indulging in processed foods, sitting for prolonged periods of time, lacking a routine, or not drinking enough water. The bigger the change, the more the reptilian part of the brain will look for the worst-case scenario and find hundreds of excuses to avoid doing the uncomfortable. So, we procrastinate, postpone, get obsessed with details. In principle, we do anything to stay in the comfort zone and avoid realizing our plans.

The most common approach to personal transformation is to make a radical change and try to hold onto the new lifestyle. Going vegan is a good example, or starting to train for a marathon with no prior running experience. And therein lies the problem: while making a big change sounds inspiring at the moment, it often ends in failure, frustration, or burnout. That change is so disruptive to the usual lifestyle that the mind resists it with all its force. Small changes, on the other hand, are often more powerful than the big ones, because they are sustainable. They are invisible from day to day but accumulated over time transform the lifestyle and take it to a whole new level. It is called continuous improvement: slowly and slightly adjusting our normal everyday habits and behaviors to form those big, radical changes.

A "vehicle pull" is one of the most spectacular parts of a strongman competition. If you haven't seen it, imagine a person pulling a heavy vehicle, typically a truck, a bus, or even a plane, across a short course (around 100ft or 30 meters) with only the power of his body. Watching from the side, it seems like an impossible task, as the strongmen struggle to get moving. It takes a colossal effort and several fierce individual pulls to get the vehicle going, but once rolling, the weight of the vehicle starts to work for it and makes the job of the strongman easier. Which of the pulls made the vehicle move? The answer: every one of them. Each of the small efforts added together created momentum that ultimately carried it across the line. The same works in life. Most of the things we achieve are the result of small changes repeated consistently.

Leading an active lifestyle and being energized on a daily basis is not something unachievable or ambiguous. **Instead, it's a combination of small healthy practices, a series of steps taken one after the other that make us better.** Not perfect, just better: even by as little as 1%.[1] We can always find something that we can improve in our life, a small action we can do, activity we can take part in, or a healthy behavior we can adopt that supports high performance. That one small change is all that we really need to build an active and healthy lifestyle. Do it consistently: one healthy activity followed by another, and over time it will compound and create a snowball effect. Training load, lifestyle and even results that seem out of reach right now will become a standard in the future.

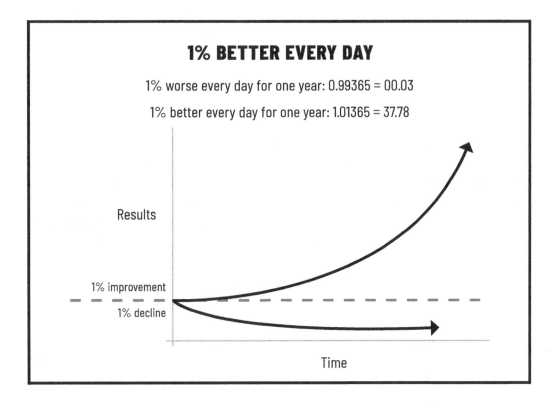

The effect of small changes. If you find a way to become just 1% better every day, compounded over time it will make you almost 38 times better a year from now.

----

1   In reference to the 1% better concept every day, introduced by James Clear in his book "Atomic Habits: An Easy and Proven Way to Build Good Habits and Break Bad Ones".

Living a healthy and active lifestyle spreads beyond just performance and into every area of life. Once we stop letting our instincts guide us and take consistent intelligent action, the planning part of our brain starts to take over. Every accomplishment, big or small, triggers a release of the hormone called dopamine that makes us experience pleasure and satisfaction. So, as we accumulate momentum with each small success, we generate more pleasure and feel more motivated to do something that we haven't done before. That effect triggers positive change across all areas of life, which is why we tend to aim higher and get excited when we have achieved something. And when we lead an active lifestyle, we don't only improve our physical performance, but also bring our better self to relationships, work or even business.

Motivation will follow if you have the guts to go without it.

When we have created momentum, any positive behavior we want to cultivate becomes automatic. Every small change to the lifestyle has the opportunity to become a habit and grow into a massive force that helps an individual achieve what he or she desires. Now that you are an athlete, you should think like one. Ask yourself: Is what I'm doing on a daily basis helping me become the best version of myself? What would an athlete do instead? How can I improve myself and my lifestyle by just 1%?"

HOW TO BUILD A SUSTAINABLE LIFESTYLE?

At a first glance, leading an active and healthy lifestyle might seem intimidating. Waking up early, exercising, watching over your diet, meditating, it all sounds like too much work, right? But it's not that complicated. All one needs to do is develop a few good habits and the rest will take care of itself.

When I had just started working in the office, I often experienced headaches towards the end of the day. It was a pulsating pain at the back of my head that seemed to occur randomly. At some point in time, however, I noticed that the headache tends to appear in the second half of the workday and, in particular, after I have had a few snacks. After reading about how dehydration and refined sugars cause energy and mood swings, as an experiment I tried substituting sugary snacks with fruits and nuts and increasing my water intake. That simple change has not only removed headaches, but also made me feel more energetic throughout the day. And the snowball kept rolling. Next I tried going to bed early to get more sleep and recover for training sessions. Surprisingly, that led to me waking up early and having time for a morning run and meditating. I continued to play around with other small habits only to discover a lifestyle that was much healthier than I ever thought I could manage.

Changing habits or developing new ones is not a quick process and it requires patience, discipline, and persistence. Sometimes a habit is a result of a deeper issue (i.e., emotional) that requires work on self-awareness and regulation first, but it doesn't require an "all or nothing" attitude to make a change in life. Just getting started is good enough. Often, making a change in one area of life creates a domino effect and puts in motion the process of self-transformation.

This section will introduce the framework for continuously improving and transforming the lifestyle, while the remaining chapters in this part of the book will breakdown the athlete's lifestyle further. Use the healthy practices from the chapters ahead to discover what actions and habits you can implement in your daily life to create that snowball effect and become more resilient.

FIND THE LEAD DOMINO

The "Domino Effect" of lifestyle change entails that a shift in one behavior can trigger a chain reaction and affect other behaviors or habits as well. Which is why the first step in enabling personal transformation and creating an active lifestyle is to determine what action will have the most positive impact on as many life areas as possible.

Take waking up an hour earlier, for example. It is a simple action, but how much positive change it can bring. It frees up time for training, meditation, journaling, practicing hobbies, spending uninterrupted time with family, and working on personal projects. Not to mention that it requires going to bed earlier, which leaves no room for late-night snacking and binge-watching TV shows. Just imagine how your health, relationships, motivation, and life satisfaction will be affected by this one change?

This is a great time to revisit the 5 Why strategy introduced in Chapter 2. Discover what behaviors are not working for you, as well as their root cause, and think of habits and automations you can introduce to turn them around.

Ask yourself:

- What one thing I can do that would make everything else easier?
- What am I doing or not doing that's holding me back?
- What's stopping me from giving my absolute best?
- What should I stop doing to start changing and what can I do instead?

BREAK THE HABIT DOWN TO THE SMALLEST ACTIVITY

A black and white thinking pattern is when we tell ourselves, '*I am either all in or I pass.*' When getting in shape requires an annual gym membership, a fancy bike or at least a new trendy outfit, otherwise it's not serious. When eating healthier means jumping on a Paleo/Keto/Atkins diet or even going full vegan because if it's not a radical shift, it doesn't count. Such an all or nothing mindset is nothing more than a search for the winning strategy which does not exist.

Big life and behavioral changes can be very intimidating, especially if there are many of them at once. It's much less stressful to focus on something small. Build your lifestyle one habit at a time and make it as easy as possible for yourself by splitting it into a series of small steps.

- Before getting on a restrictive diet or manipulating your carbs/fats/protein ratio to "lose weight," start by simply adding more healthy ingredients into your meals (i.e., leafy greens, vegetables, legumes), and eating less sugary and processed foods.

- Before embarking on a high intensity transformational program to "get in shape," discipline yourself to do a form of exercise for 30 minutes every day for a month.

- Before pushing yourself through a detox to "cleanse the body" start by drinking 2L of water daily and cutting out alcohol, coffee and added sugar for a week.

- Before experimenting with fasting (intermittent or prolonged fasts) start by cutting out fast-food (including takeaway coffee and treats) for a week.

- Before buying a range of nutritional supplements to "improve recovery and reduce mental stress" start by getting consistent 8 hours of sleep per night for more than a week.

- Before buying an annual gym membership do bodyweight exercises (pushups, lunges, squats, pullups, planks, etc.) at home 3–4 times per week for 30 seconds each with little rest in between.

MASTER THE ART OF SHOWING UP

One of the most effective ways to make a good habit stick is to become great at starting something. Be it exercising, eating a more nutritious diet, or following a daily schedule. Once you make the activity ridiculously easy to begin (break the habit down), practice starting until it becomes a habit. You don't need to make it perfect, just get yourself going. For example, if you want to start running, flipping through an athlete's social media feed or watching an inspiring movie will not get you to the start line of a marathon. Putting on running shoes and going for a 10 min run will. Once out the door, you will notice that all excuses fade away and that initial resistance dissipates.

Quitting before we even tried something is a common form of limitation that we put on ourselves. And that behavior is amplified every time we make an excuse not to do something. '*I can't wake up early because I'm not a morning person. I can't make healthy meals because I'm bad at cooking. I can't go running because it's raining.*' We can never know where our true limits are without trying. And even when we think we know, those limits can always be pushed. Whenever we tell ourselves I can't, that's our cue to do that thing we're trying to avoid—as hard as it may be.

The struggle to do something new is always the hardest when we begin. **But once we start something, more often than not, it gets easier to carry on.** Like getting out the door to start the run or getting in the car to drive to the gym. In fact, completing that first action provides a little shot of dopamine that generates pleasure. We feel good about the fact that despite resistance, we did get ourselves off the couch and out the door. Just like pulling a heavy vehicle, the more momentum we gain the easier it gets. Those internal battles that we have in our brain will always be there; they don't go away. We just get better at choosing what's right for us.

STRATEGY: ALWAYS DO THE WARM-UP

Athletes know very well that lack of energy and low motivation is very subjective and can often be deceiving. More often than not, those lethargic feelings are nothing more than mental resistance manifested through the physical body. A good practice that athletes use to get over this hurdle is committing to always completing a warmup before deciding about skipping a session.

Warm-ups are a very important component of the training process. They increase the core body temperature, promote blood circulation to deliver oxygen and nutrients to the muscles and brain quicker, and remove any muscle tightness which might slow down that blood flow. All of it sets the body up for better performance by extending time to fatigue, improving power and speed, and boosting energy and focus. Besides that, when athletes go through the usual motions to get ready for the session, they switch their focus to a "different frequency" and tune in to the present moment, which helps to get in the right mood. If after that, the body still feels under-recovered, then it makes sense to take the session easy or take a break.

It's the same in life—any great performance will need some warming up. If you feel stuck, low on energy or struggling with motivation, just start somewhere and focus on the next immediate action. Don't make judgements on how you feel about a particular activity or action before you begin. Appearance can be deceiving, and we can never know exactly how the body feels and whether it is ready for a session until we go for it. We can never know if we have the inspiration or the drive to do something until we try it. They say the best runs are those that almost didn't happen, and the most satisfying achievements are those where we almost gave up. Focus on starting; don't think too much about how you'll finish. If you put in the work, the finish will come eventually.

BUILD DISCIPLINE THROUGH AUTOMATIONS

Motivation to do something is temporary. It comes and goes, like the sun in the cloudy sky on a windy October day. We tend to be very motivated when the sun is shining and everything is perfect when we're fully rested, when there's little stress, when we and those closest to us are well and happy. However, once the clouds of adversity or fatigue get in the way, the sunshine is gone and with that the motivation to make something happen.

Relying on motivation or willpower to make healthy choices in life is not very sustainable. Those are finite resources and can change based on multitude of factors, including sleep or hunger. We start every day with a certain amount of juice in our mental batteries (willpower) and "consume" it throughout the day. Our reptilian brain likes comfort, so as we get more tired or stressed, making healthy choices becomes increasingly difficult. As a result, we become more likely to procrastinate important decisions and actions, get addicted to something or revert to convenient, but unhealthy food options.

People don't quit on day 20 of the 30-day challenge or abandon their New Year's resolutions in July. They tend to quit when the hard work begins—when the excitement of starting something new wanes off and the daily grind takes over. Even the best motivational speech in the world can only ignite a temporary spark. It will not change a person's life unless he or she builds discipline around it.

What makes the habit stick, be it good or bad, is **automation**. Regardless of whether you want to develop good habits or stop the bad ones, a system is much more powerful than willpower. And it's not that complicated to implement. All that is required is to reduce the complexity of a good habit and increase it for the bad one. That will make the desired behavior the easiest one to do.

Here are some examples:

- Put your phone in the next room while working. That way, you won't be distracted by all notifications.
- Lay out running clothes the evening before, so once you put them on in the morning it's much easier to get out the door.
- Put a timer on your router to switch off the internet at 10PM to give ample time to wind down before bed.

STRATEGY: DON'T SKIP TWO IN A ROW

Leading a healthy lifestyle or following a training program is not an all-or-nothing endeavor. We're all humans and none of us is perfect. Everyone makes mistakes and there is always a chance to face circumstances under which our healthy habits or training schedule are put at risk. However, it's never one mistake that derails the whole plan or lifestyle. It's almost always a series of slip-offs that create a downward spiral.

One mistake is not a big deal, unless it creates frustration about not being perfect. Feeling bad about missing a day of training or engaging in negative self-talk after having a cheat meal makes it more likely to make a misstep the next time. Then it's even more likely we miss the third time, kind of like thinking, "*I'm losing anyway, so what's the point of trying.*" Even professional athletes don't follow their prescribed program fully and skip some of the workouts. The same goes for good lifestyle habits, the behaviors we repeat consistently, but not necessarily perfectly. Discipline is about how we are able to pull ourselves together and recover from these individual slip-offs.

Break the pattern before it even comes up. Not skipping 2 in a row means compensating for that initial mistake with a positive action. For example, if you missed a training session, don't beat yourself up for it. Just make sure you don't miss the next one and carry on with the plan. If you had a cheat meal, make sure you drink a healthy smoothie as a snack later on to get back on track. This simple strategy is very effective at ensuring consistency, be it in training, healthy eating or any other habit we are building.

The all-or-nothing approach is a big factor for why many New Year's resolutions fail. Discipline isn't always about perfection sometimes it's only about showing up. It's OK to slow down, but once we fully stop it's really hard to get the momentum back.

THE MONTHLY CHALLENGE: DAILY EXERCISE

The challenges presented in this part of the book are designed to push you to get your lifestyle to the next level. They sound simple at first, but also, they break your existing routine, which is exactly what makes them effective. Embrace the discomfort and take small consistent action to make your lifestyle work for you—one step at a time.

I strongly believe that if you want to become good at something, you have to practice it often. Real and sustainable results come from daily work that requires discipline and consistent good habits: not three days per week, not when you feel like it, but every single day. Physical fitness is no exception. Frequency is the secret sauce of every top athlete, as consistent easy exercise gradually builds strength and endurance across the entire body. Over time, that habit creates a snowball effect making performance that seems out of reach for most people feel nearly effortless for an athlete. Many Tour de France riders share how they feel a little off following a day without cycling. So, on a rest day they prefer to do a light spin of 1–2 hours as active recovery.

The single best thing a person can do for his or her fitness is to move every day as much as possible and do it in various ways. Riding a bike, running, hiking, or even taking a Yoga or Pilates class. Movement is life and the more we challenge our body, the more adaptations we trigger. As a result, the more resilient it becomes. On top of that, light activity stimulates blood flow (see Chapter 10) which generates the energy to follow healthy behaviors and put in the effort in other areas of life as well.

THE 30/30 CHALLENGE

Commit to a minimum of thirty minutes of daily activity for the next thirty days. It doesn't have to be anything specific or even a hard session for that matter—a hike, a yoga or Pilates class, or a bodyweight workout would be sufficient. However, it does have to be an organized daily exercise. Block that time in your planner or calendar and show up. Every day, upon completing the practice, check it off the list.

When it feels difficult to include a training session in your daily schedule or you feel low on energy, remind yourself that it is only for thirty days. Then, think about how it will feel someday when you are out there living the adventure.

Increase your odds of success by adding external accountability to your challenge. Post your intent and progress on social media with hashtags #resilientathlete and #trainforadventure.

PAYING ATTENTION
TO YOUR BODY

There is never a good time to be injured or get sick. Exam period, deadlines, stressful projects at work, upcoming competitions, or even a vacation in a foreign land. Being sidelined always seems to happen at the worst possible time. In fact, athletes in their peak form or going into competitions are usually at the greatest risk of catching a cold or a virus. Some (like me) even twice. Strange, isn't it? Shouldn't training make people stronger and healthier, not feeling worse?

It was the summer before I started university and I was in an intense training block in preparation for the European Championships. I was putting a lot of energy into training that year and my fitness was the best it had ever been. Things looked very promising until just over a month before the race. A virus forced me to stop training and spend 10 days in bed with a high fever and intense throat pain that made it very difficult to eat or drink. Once back on my feet I didn't take any time to reflect. Instead I jumped right back into training as soon as possible with the goal to get my fitness back while there was still time. A week later, another virus, two more weeks in bed and zero progress. While it felt sudden at the moment, the body did send clear warning signals. I simply chose to treat them as something I had to "muscle" through. Waking up sweating from the afternoon nap, constant fatigue, and poor times during speed intervals—the body was clearly under tremendous stress, so it started pulling all the plugs to get me to take the break which it desperately needed.

When we don't allow our body to recover sufficiently, we start to accumulate stress. The hormone cortisol decreases the level of white blood cells, which reduces the body's ability to defend itself. As a result, it grows weaker and loses the ability to fight off bacteria and infections. It also takes much longer to heal wounds and recover in general. In moderation, stress is actually a good thing because after a short recovery, we adapt and grow stronger. The line between being fit and becoming ill or injured is very thin and sometimes it's pushed too far.

> *Injury or illness happens when we disconnect from our bodies and focus too much on the external world—expectations, goals, competition—instead of what is best for ourselves and our bodies.*

We do have a great natural defense system capable of protecting us from many illnesses and injuries, but leading an unhealthy lifestyle has the power to sabotage it over time. Unbalanced and unhealthy nutrition, lousy sleep habits, stressful environment, not to mention the hardcore training regime. All of it puts our bodies under a lot of pressure and weakens the immune system. What's more, ambitions, excitement, and expectations often force athletes to ignore the warning signs (pain or fatigue) and push the body to do more than it can handle. Becoming ill or suffering an injury is our body's natural way of saying "hey, slow down, take a moment and reconsider what you're doing." Injury or illness happens for a reason, so instead of fighting it, use it to become more resilient in the future.

Everybody is different and none of us receives a personalized manual that explains exactly what we are capable of, how quickly we can recover, or what we should do to improve. But it doesn't mean we have to go to war with ourselves, say, "Shut up, legs" and push until exhaustion. A more sustainable approach is to use intelligent testing: instead of muting the signals that the body sends, use them to self-direct fitness. Give the body what it needs at the moment, not what we expect it to deliver. Often, that requires taking a step back or taking things easy. Is everything really on track? Am I training too hard? Am I managing the overall stress? Am I eating the right foods to support performance and the immune system?

The secret to achieving extraordinary results is to listen to yourself. In sports, it is listening to your body. In everyday life, it's listening to your ideas and staying true to your vision. Everyone has their own pace and it's important to create a lifestyle that elevates it and generates energy instead of wasting it. Resilient athletes live in the moment—they don't overthink things. They train on feel, eat foods that nourish them, and do it all with joy and an admirable degree of humility. Behind that exterior, it is a very intentional human—an athlete with the drive to test the very limits of human capability and become the best version of him or herself.

Tuning in with the body is about understanding all the factors that caused or might cause a specific response. By doing that, we can find ways to optimize our life and have more energy for the things that matter whether it is practicing hobbies, being present with family or even training more. We can prevent and minimize the negative effects (pain, fatigue), while maximizing the positive ones (feeling energetic and strong). Doing so starts with becoming mindful of our own body.

BECOME YOUR OWN DETECTIVE

It's not uncommon for people to be ignorant to the signals that the body sends. In fact, more often than not, those are muted, buried under the layers of "more important" things that are going on in life. An occasional headache, a dry mouth, sporadic knee pain, or even shortness of breath while climbing stairs. What is often written off as a minor inconvenience might be an indicator that something's off or is on a negative trajectory. Athletes tend to be more sensitive to these physiological sensations thanks to the special bond they have developed with their bodies over countless hours of practice: the mind-body connection.

But not every athlete puts his or her long-term health over short-term performance. There's this notion that whoever engages in physical exercise should be bulletproof and show no signs of weakness in order to become better—kind of a "fake it till you make it" approach. **Needless to say, that in this mindset, it is easy for an athlete to overlook a key link in the performance chain and take training a bit too far.** And this prioritization is not something that only amateur athletes struggle with. Sometimes even top athletes begin to recognize the value of tuning in with the body too late, usually after a certain illness or injury has already sidelined them.

There's a running joke among physical therapists that "there are two types of athletes: those who have been injured and those who will be." And just like in any joke there's a large element of truth in it. If we do not take care of our body and pay attention to the warning signals, it will eventually force us to take a break. Any athlete who has been injured is eager not to repeat the situation of being unable to practice for a prolonged period of time. So, often after a particularly disturbing experience, there's awareness about what to look for so an athlete starts to pay attention to how the body feels. He or she develops sensitivity to various aches and pains and through that, learns how the body responds to various training loads. Sometimes that's all they need to stop training through the pain and instead be vigilant and proactively look for ways to minimize the possibility of injury induced downtime in the future. Even a minor pain is a signal that something is off, and you should correct it instead of ignoring it.

I had many experiences that put me out of training and competing. Accidents aside, injuries and illnesses felt conceptually the same. I pushed myself beyond what was comfortable, weakened the body and immune system, and that has set the scene for illness to develop or injury to occur. As frustrating as they were, each experience has helped me understand that being sidelined is not a badge of honor or a confirmation that I am pushing the limits hard enough. All it did was prevent me from going after what I really wanted. So, over time I became my own detective with the goal of proactively investigating how my body functions best. To understand which factors affect it, and how I can optimize my lifestyle and the environment to put myself in the best position to reach my goals.

The body doesn't come with a user manual, and neither are we born with knowledge of the exact ingredients needed to become the best version of ourselves: what to do, how far to push or how long to rest. However, being your own detective and tuning in to your body helps you to discover that recipe. To become more aware of the cues that the body sends, better understand what it needs most and what it's capable of at every moment, and even to tell the difference between hunger, thirst, tiredness, and emotional distress. Gradually, that mind-body connection will begin to influence our everyday life by means of healthier decisions. For example, instead of reaching for a candy bar or another sugary snack when tired, we'll be able to reach for a glass of water, take a mindfulness break or even give ourselves permission to take a nap instead of pushing through the fatigue, reduce the intensity of the training session or take a rest day.

The best part about knowing how the body responds to specific factors is the power it gives to influence the training process. **A training plan is only as good as its execution.** It doesn't make sense to follow the plan of an elite marathoner only to find yourself fatigued and skipping sessions within a couple of weeks. Experienced athletes know exactly what works for them and, therefore, can focus on it. They tend to shift their training sessions to maximize recovery and get the maximum benefit. Tailoring a plan in that way allows them to keep it optimized and avoid unnecessary fatigue. This way they can include more quality training sessions and, ultimately, get better results.

Understanding what the body is communicating helps to make healthier choices that compound over time and lead to greater health and emotional well-being.

In the academic world, it's called interoceptive awareness: the ability to identify, understand, and respond appropriately to the patterns of internal signals. Colloquially, it's called tuning in with the body which means the expertise of an athlete to recognize how he or she feels based on personal markers or bodily sensations (like breathing, heart rate, fatigue, muscle tension, etc.) and make an informed decision about the best course of action. However, it doesn't end with training. Instead, when such recognition takes place, things start to click and get carried over to the rest of the lifestyle, like a snowball effect. That's when athletes start to think about how the foods they eat nourish them or how their bedtime affects recovery.

A resilient athlete is a part-time detective, investigating and tracing back the steps that are required to optimize the lifestyle for high-performance, constantly thinking, *'What can I do to put myself in the best position to achieve my goals?'* We own the key to our own health, so we need to take care of it. No one else will. If you have good results and look strong on the outside, that doesn't mean the body is not heading towards crash or burnout. Befriend the idea of continuous improvement and look for every possibility to improve and optimize how your body performs. It doesn't require an injury or illness to start being mindful of different signals the body sends:

- **Start with practicing the so-called body scan.** This is a practice of bringing attention to the body and noticing various sensations, like pain, tension, numbness, feelings of relaxation or ease. Not doing anything about it, just noticing. You can even integrate this simple meditation practice into daily de-stressing rituals before going to bed. Alternatively, you can join a class or use an app that will guide you through any other body-focused mindfulness practice. Yoga would be a great choice. It's probably the most well-known and widely practiced form of body awareness exercise that uses breath and movement to become more connected with the body and mind.

- **Try not to ignore, belittle, over amplify, or judge any of the sensations you feel whether they are good or bad.** Consider it all as valuable information. People often don't know what causes a certain sensation or what contributes to injury or illness, which is why they often miss the signals that the body gives them. This is a good time to develop a journaling practice to record how the body feels and what behavior preceded the good or bad sensation. Once you know the history, you will be in a better position to recognize the unhealthy behavior and limit it.

- **Work on developing your perspective by analyzing what has caused a particular sensation and what effect it can have on you.** For example, having a dry mouth could be a result of not hydrating well throughout the day or a signal that the body is under a lot of stress due to the daily workouts you have been doing. Either way, such dehydration means that any physical activity will be more intense than planned and might require more recovery time. By having such context instead of simply ignoring the sensation, athletes put themselves in a position to make decisions about their training and lifestyle that elevates their fitness, not only creates fatigue.

STRATEGY: TRAINING DIARY

You can develop the skill of listening to your body by means of keeping a training log or a diary. It can be a simple notebook, or even an online spreadsheet, whatever is easier for you to maintain. Besides training data (like duration, heart rate, what was done), record the specifics of how you feel on a daily basis. How you slept, what you ate, if there is ease or any tightness in the body—the more details the better.

When you review this data after the session or several weeks later, you will start to identify various patterns in your lifestyle. Things like low quality sleep after a large dinner or night out, joint stiffness after an extensive strength training, or feeling energized after a recovery session. All of these data points are opportunities to optimize the lifestyle and training process and tailor those specifically to you.

A training diary helps to spot areas needing improvement, but it also works as a reference for past good performances. For example, what factors led to a personal best in a race or a particularly good feeling in a training session? Most of what athletes do gets repeated on a consistent basis—training, recovery, nutrition, or racing. Having notes to look back at to see what has worked well (i.e., warm up, nutrition, recovery, race strategy) is very helpful. This reference allows the athlete to replicate a good performance and avoid repeating a bad one. It is what they call an athlete's experience.

Personally, when I look back at my competitive career, I realize that this simple practice of recording my progress forced me to consistently reflect on what was going well and what did not. Over time, it kept me focused and improved the quality of my training sessions. Moreover, whenever I returned to focused training after a longer break or trained for a new adventure reviewing my training logs always helped me to discover patterns: what has worked well and where I took it too far. Guiding my training and lifestyle in such a way is a major factor helping me stay motivated and energized to train even more.

LISTEN TO YOUR HEART

While chatting with fellow athletes after one of the sessions on my first spring training camp, I learned that their coach asks them to wear a strange device during training. It was 2005 and the words, "heart rate monitor," was not yet on everyone's lips. I had no idea what was that strap they put around their chest or why it was needed. But I was eager to learn, so I approached the coach to find out. For someone in his late 50s he was surprisingly versed in the new technology at the time that was heart rate training. He shared that the purpose of the heart rate monitor is for him to see how well his athletes execute training programs and how their bodies respond to the workload, and how adjusting the training load to fit the athlete's current condition leads to better and more sustainable results. The lesson he gave me that afternoon stayed with me for my entire sports career, even though I didn't understand it right away "it takes a lot of mental strength to push yourself to the limit, but it's much harder to know when to pull back."

To say I was intrigued would be an understatement. The gadget geek in me was ecstatic, and an ambitious teenager saw an opportunity. Until then, I only had an on/off switch and thought you go hard in training and repeat the next day, for as long as you can maintain. I compared myself with others and tried to replicate or "beat" them in every training session, which mostly left me tired, over-trained and frustrated from not seeing desired results. My attention was all over the place. In fact, the only place it wasn't at was my body. Interoceptive awareness, mind-body connection and body intelligence might as well have been words in a foreign language because to me they made no sense.

But that was about to change.

I purchased my first heart rate monitor within a few months of returning from that training camp, and it became my guide in the world of self-discovery. Since the day that I first put on that chest strap, I tracked my heart rate daily, before, during and after sessions. I sometimes even went to bed wearing it to find out what my average heart rate was during sleep. Using heart rate in training gradually improved results from my efforts. It was very useful to know what to focus on and I was able to bring more quality to the training process through controlling the intensity and keeping track of my recovery. In particular, I noticed that in most cases what I thought was a 70% effort was closer to 90%, because I got carried away competing with others. By no means was it a quick process, but over time, I learned how my body responds to stress, what effect different intensities and training sessions have on me and, ultimately, how training programs should be designed, adjusted and executed.

During times of higher stress, physical, psychological or environmental, the body has to work harder. It requires more energy to move itself, supply nutrients to the muscles, support increased brain activity, process cortisol and adrenaline hormones, cool itself down, repair the damage done during the training session, even more. Sometimes it's hot and humid outside, which makes exercising harder. Sometimes we are a little under-recovered after a hard session the day before. Or maybe the body is not fully over a cold and is still fighting bacteria. All of these factors force the heart to pump more blood and result in an elevated heart rate. Paying attention to it will help to reveal the factors which the brain might ignore.

Heart rate is an athlete's best friend, during and outside training. Unlike the reptilian brain, it won't tell you what you want to hear only to justify skipping a workout and staying on the couch.

The heart rate is the best indicator of the overall levels of stress that the body is going through at the moment. Recovery activities happen in the background and continue for hours and even days after the stress response took place. We can do a high intensity sprint set or go out with friends one night, the result will be the same, an elevated heart rate the next morning. That is not a coincidence. Instead, it is a reflection of how stressed the body is and how unprepared it would be for a hard training session.

Coming fully rested for the key sessions is important for optimizing performance. That way, athletes are able to execute the session well, tolerate more training load, and improve. Which is why athletes and coaches use heart rate to organize the training process in such a way that fatigue is balanced and specific adaptations to stress are targeted.

Fatigue, mental stress, hectic lifestyle, illness, these are just some examples of factors that affect an athlete's fitness condition and, by means of that, the heart rate. However, instead of tweaking each individual factor in an attempt to optimize the energy levels and performance, there is a more effective approach. In the same way that certain intensity levels trigger specific adaptation processes in our body, certain times of day have a specific effect on our body. Optimizing the daily regime, therefore, is a lead domino that will have a lasting effect on all areas of performance.

STRATEGY: RESTING HEART RATE

Resting heart rate (Rest HR or RHR) is a measurement taken when the body is at peace. Usually, first thing in the morning, even before rolling out of bed. It serves as an indicator of the level of overall stress and is a great way to tell if the body is in optimal condition for a training session or not. By monitoring resting heart rate on a daily basis, athletes can learn how various factors affect their recovery and also time training sessions for maximum performance.

To calculate heart rate, simply put two fingers on the inner side of the wrist (closer to the thumb) or on the side of your throat (slightly below the jaw). Count how many beats your heart makes in 10 seconds and multiply that by 6.

Everyone's heart rate is individual, so it's important to establish a baseline first: an average RHR for the past seven days. An average person's RHR is typically somewhere between 60 and 90 beats per minute (bpm). Younger people and women on average tend to have slightly higher rates, whereas for trained athletes (men or women), the resting heart rate is often well below 50 bpm (especially for those practicing endurance sports). Thanks to regular aerobic exercise, the heart increases in size and the capillary network gets more developed, which leads to more blood being pumped out and transported across the body more effectively with every beat. As a result, for athletes, a decrease in heart rate over time can also be a signal of improvements in aerobic fitness.

Generally, RHR higher than ~5–7 bpm or 10% (whichever is higher) than the baseline indicates that the body is not fully recovered, and the body is under stress, be it fatigue from a hard training session or even a stressful week at work. Monitoring RHR on a daily basis will give athletes an understanding of how the recovery after a hard training session is progressing. It can also help them to notice the first signs of overtraining and be a reference in determining how quickly after an illness to resume high intensity training.

- **Training load.** If RHR on a given day is higher than the baseline (+10% or more), athletes should take a rest day or do a very easy session in Zone 1 (see Chapter 14 for more on heart rate training). By training through fatigue, athletes risk pushing the body too far and slowing down their progress. However, if RHR is elevated over a period of several weeks, then it's a signal of accumulated fatigue: the body is probably operating on reserves and slowly moving into overtraining. This is the time to consider taking a recovery week or even several days completely off.

- **Illness.** During an illness, the body temperature increases and, as a result, RHR also becomes elevated. It's estimated that for every 1°C increase, RHR can jump by as much as 10–15 bpm, because the body is working overtime to cool itself and fight disease. Athletes are generally eager to get back into training after an illness, however, resuming intense training after the first symptoms have subsided is risky. Wait for the RHR to return to baseline and only then start to include intense intervals into your schedule.

THE PERFECT DAY

Energy is our fuel: the more we have it the more capacity we have to perform and the more motivated we are to put in the effort to reach our full potential. However, if we waste energy on unnecessary or detrimental activities, our ability to perform, productivity, and even health, gets compromised. Many people know this in theory, but their lifestyle does not allow them to benefit from that knowledge. Professionals and top performers have the same level of energy as everyone else, yet they tend to achieve much more than an average person thanks to habits and routines that regulate its usage. So, what would it look like for you to be the pro version of yourself?

Imagine it is a typical Tuesday morning. You wake up at 5:30AM, fully rested, having clocked solid eight hours of sleep. Instead of jumping on social media, you do a short mobility routine, hydrate, and have a handful of dates to give you energy for your morning exercise. An hour later, you are back from an easy training practice just in time for breakfast with the family, scrambled tofu with vegetables and avocado. Protein and fats will break down slowly throughout the morning and prevent mood and energy swings. You drink herbal tea with a handful of dried fruits before heading out to drop your kids off at school and go to work.

Throughout the day, you avoid sugar and drink plenty of water instead. You have planned ahead and done meal prep, which means you have a homemade smoothie as a mid-morning snack, protein-based lunch, and an afternoon snack. At work, you are fully awake and present, not only for your ten o'clock meeting, but also for the presentation you have at one, right after lunch.

Roughly two hours before finishing work, you have a carb-rich meal to give you the energy to complete the intense session you have planned. The timing is no accident: it's intentionally integrated into the schedule to ensure you get a good workout in. You have all of your gear in the car, so once you close the laptop, you drive to the nearest park and do a 40-minute session there that includes sets of two or three minute intense intervals with an equal walking break in between.

You eat a handful of dried fruits on your way home to help your body start the recovery processes. Upon arriving, you take a shower starting with warm water and turn it gradually to cold after a few minutes. It's unpleasant at first, so you breathe deeply and once the body adapts, it almost feels good. Once you step out of the shower, you feel completely rejuvenated and wide awake. You spend a few minutes foam rolling the muscles before an early dinner of coconut lentil curry with rice and cooked vegetables that keeps you full up until bedtime. It's a busy yet rewarding day and there's still an entire evening ahead to spend with the family.

Turns out you can live the life of a pro athlete and train 10+ hours per week while still having a family and a day job, eating in a consistent way, and overall, having a life. Doing so might sound like a lot of boxes to tick. But if we look closely, there's nothing in it that a regular person is not already doing—family, work, training, sleep, cooking, eating. It is all just a little more organized. The best part about it is that such an optimized lifestyle not only elevates physical performance, but also has a positive effect on mental health. Accomplishing more throughout the day and doing what you are passionate about brings joy and happiness. Being organized about it helps to minimize the feeling of lethargy and become energized instead. And it all starts with establishing the daily regime.

How many times have you thought it would be great to do something, but you felt you just didn't have the energy for it? **The truth is, the majority of us have the ability to optimize our lives to use less energy, so that they can spend it on training, recovery and adding more exciting things into life.** You might have heard already about circadian rhythms: physical, mental, and behavioral patterns that follow a 24-hour cycle. Our body also has an internal clock, and it carries out certain essential functions and processes at specific times of day. Waking up and falling asleep, regulating body temperature, releasing certain hormones and so on. These processes happen automatically, without our active involvement and are preceded by certain signals, like feeling sleepy or hungry at specific times of day. Studies found that athletic performance can vary over the course of the day by up to 26%, depending on the athlete's circadian rhythm.[1]

However, when circadian rhythms are disrupted then signals from the body's internal clock subside and it requires more energy to operate effectively.

---

1   According to the 2015 research paper titled "The Impact of Circadian Phenotype and Time since Awakening on Diurnal Performance in Athletes" published in the journal *Current Biology*.

Picture yourself in a busy foreign city. Let's say you're in New York and you want to go out for a run. You might have taken a look at the map and planned a route to follow. That first run will require a lot of mental energy, looking at the street names to find the right one that gets you to that promenade you want, navigating construction works and closed streets, maybe even peeking at the map in your smartphone to make sure you are on track. Then there's always the challenge of finding the way back. Those first few runs in a foreign place are always stressful, but every next time, you can cover the same route with less thinking because you know what to expect. Now imagine if the body needed to make those small decisions for every little activity we do on a daily basis. It would start to calm itself down and get ready to sleep only after we are in bed, which means we would have to lay there for hours until the nervous system relaxes. Or it would start producing hormones that regulate the digestive system only after we had eaten, leaving us bloated and sleepy after a meal. This is what happens when circadian rhythms are disrupted as a result of the lack of schedule for the body to follow. It cannot optimize itself, so every process takes longer or requires more energy to complete.

There is a way to "reset" circadian rhythms and make them work for us, not against. Start with developing a regular sleep schedule: go to bed and wake up at the same time every day. This will help the body to establish a pattern to follow and gradually become more energized throughout the day. Don't just stop there. The timing of what we do also matters. **If we align our activities with what the body is most optimized to do at certain times of day, we will be more effective at them and have more energy to spare.**

If that sounds too complicated, don't worry. Luckily, nature has thought it through and actually made things pretty easy for us. The body's internal clock is regulated by the environment and, to a large extent, by the exposure to light and dark. Processes that take place in our bodies and the signals it sends us are largely determined by the phase of movement of the sun. That influence is very strong and unless we lock ourselves in a closed space with artificial lighting and no windows, we can do little about it. Have you ever been on an overnight camping trip and caught yourself feeling sleepy soon after sunset? The invention of electricity and artificial lighting doesn't mean we are no longer influenced by nature, it just means that the body has a harder time adjusting to a more demanding or hectic lifestyle.

In other words, the sun and the amount of light determines the flow of energy in our body. Once we recognize this connection, it becomes possible to optimize our lifestyle for more energy. In fact, we can even improve our performance by connecting with nature in such a way. By coordinating activities with our natural circadian rhythms, and all of it starts with waking up early. That one habit has a direct impact on the quality of energy we get in life.

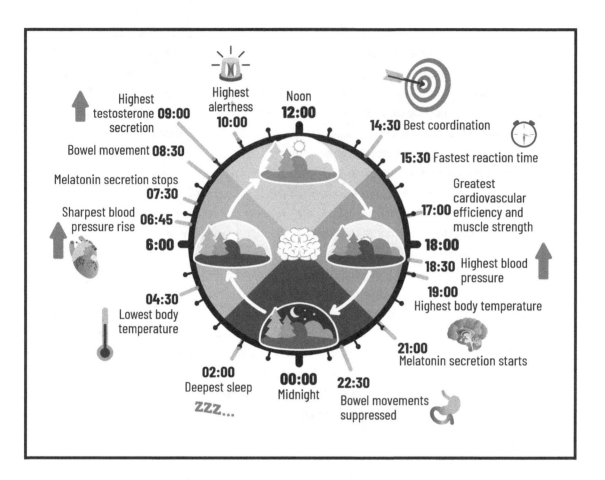

The effect of natural circadian rhythms depending on the position of the sun.[1]

---

1   In reference to the work of Michael Smolensky and Lynne Lamberg in their book *The Body Clock Guide to Better Health: How to Use your Body's Natural Clock to Fight Illness and Achieve Maximum Health.*

Morning (5AM–11AM)

There is a lot of debate on why someone should wake up early when it is also possible to do everything in the evening as well. However, it is hard to find a successful person whose career depends on consistently performing and being at the top of his or her game who sleeps in. More often than not, these top performers are overflowing with creative energy, enthusiasm and feel a sense of joy from the process. They can't wait to wake up in the morning to get going, as they seem to subconsciously understand the wisdom of the old proverb "Early to bed and early to rise makes a man healthy, wealthy, and wise." On the other hand, the less happy a person is, the higher the chance he or she would sleep more and, in that way, avoid the not so pleasing reality.

From a physiological perspective, in the early hours of the morning, our blood pressure rises, and melatonin secretion slows down, which lowers the quality of sleep we get. It is as if nature is urging us to wake up and get a jump start on the day. Have you had a situation when you were more fresh and alert after sleeping 4–5 hours than after sleeping 10? It was probably when you had to wake up earlier than usual, compared to when you had time to sleep in. A low quality of sleep provides little recovery because the body is, essentially, awake.

Moreover, after a night of sleep, our mind is fresh and free from the noise, which helps us focus better, be it on our personal projects, meditation or simply getting organized. The amount of energy our working memory can use (willpower) is limited, so we cannot focus and make decisions indefinitely. Once we use up our "decision capacity," we resist making any decision and either ignore the situation or act impulsively (resort to habits). What often happens due to waking up late is that this peaceful time becomes quite hasty. So much needs to be done with so little time. You have to get up, decide what to eat for breakfast, what to wear, pack, etc. No wonder so many people dread the experience. All of these decisions and activities build up a lot of stress that ultimately drains the willpower and sets a rushed mood for the day.

Willpower is a muscle that can be trained—the more you use it to overcome difficulties, the stronger it gets. The simple act of pushing yourself to wake up early every morning does exactly that—every time you do is a small win that reinforces good practice.

If you're like many people, going to bed around midnight and waking up with just enough time to make it to work, try to live more in accordance with natural circadian rhythms. Start by shifting the two "unproductive" hours between 10p.m. and midnight to the morning (6AM to 8AM) and use that as your personal time. Do whatever you always postpone or have no time or energy for whether that is exercise, cooking for the week, planning, or working on your personal projects. What's the alternative, anyway? Scrolling through social media before going to bed? Reading clickbait stories or watching videos designed to attract and keep your attention resulting in an endless negative loop? Shortly after you start waking up early and using that time for yourself, you will notice that you are feeling less stressed throughout the day and generally in a better mood. That's because you already did all of the important (personal) stuff early in the morning and are more relaxed about whatever the day will bring.

STRATEGY: MORNING ROUTINE

We lose control of the day the moment we hit the snooze button. Or peek into our phone first thing in the morning. Once we do that, we let the day define us instead of asking ourselves, 'What do I want to focus on?' we start the day by asking the world, 'What do others want me to focus on?'

When we prepare for an important race, we pay attention to every single detail. We get up early to eat breakfast 3 hours before the start; leave enough time for a good warm-up; organize our gear and do tons of other small things. Everything is done with the purpose of putting our body and mind into the best possible condition to deliver our best performance. However, we rarely bring our best selves to each and every day. Why don't we give ourselves enough time every day to set us up for that perfect day?

The world's most successful people don't hit the snooze button. They hop right out of bed and begin creating energy they need to make the most of every single minute of the day. They get started when most are still asleep. The trick to creating a healthy lifestyle and becoming your best self is to fall in love with the morning and give yourself plenty of time to start the day right. There is no better time to prepare the brain and the body to perform at the highest level. A morning routine in this process is like a pilot's checklist. It helps to set the entire day for success, so plan your morning as you would plan your day or week, in a way that when it comes down to it, you know exactly what to do.

By pushing yourself to wake up early and do something meaningful, you are already winning, over laziness and resistance. You will start cultivating that winner's mindset and getting more resilient with every morning. A common question is what you do when you wake up that early. The answer? Everything you postpone in the evenings. If you find it hard to wake up, plan something exciting in the morning.

Here are a few ideas to include in your morning routine:

- **Warm up and exercise.** The best way to stay consistent with training is to do it first thing in the morning. There's always a high chance that something will come up during the day, whereas in the morning, it is done and dusted.

- **Meditation.** Focusing on what you want to achieve helps to set the scene for the day and start it right. In addition to that, practicing meditation in the morning improves the skill much faster.

- **Breathing practice.** Breathing is a skill that can both calm down and energize the body. Consistent practice can help to improve control over emotional state and overall well-being.

- **Journaling and planning.** Both of these activities are great at creating change in life but require "empty space," time when you have no commitments and do not need to do something.

- **Self-development.** Early morning is the time to find what inspires you, what your purpose is, and where you can improve. There is no more excuse for not having enough time—it's about what priority you put on yourself.

As much as good habits energize us, there are some that only drain energy and attention. External stimulants that do not let us start the day on our terms and are best to be avoided, are reading emails, checking social media, watching TV (except self-development programs), or watching/reading the news in the morning.

Afternoon (11AM–5PM)

Afternoon is the time when the body is optimized for performance—blood pressure is up, coordination, reaction time, and cardiovascular endurance and strength are at their peaks. All systems are ready to go, which is why it makes sense to schedule the key training session at this point of time, or sometimes even two (at 11AM and 4PM, for instance). The body will be able to perform better, tolerate more training load, and improve more.

Besides training, there's one more area to consider for optimal lifestyle—nutrition. When we eat is as important as what we eat. Our metabolism is the fastest during daytime and it's much easier to digest food when the body is the most active. Which is why it's best to eat the biggest meal of the day during or around midday when the sun is at its highest point. It will get digested quickly and will not interfere with recovery.

Evening (5PM–10PM)

At midnight, the sun is at its lowest point and the body should be in the state of maximum relaxation to provide the best recovery. Going to bed earlier (before 10PM) ensures we do not only get more sleep and have the opportunity to wake up earlier, but also improves the quality of it thanks to melatonin secretion that starts at 9PM.

In the evenings, physical activity usually slows down, whereas mental activity not necessarily. Which is why in the evening, it is important to take it easy, wind down and relax. Prepare the body for going to bed by reducing screen time and intense brain activity. That includes minimizing scrolling through social media and watching TV. Mental exhaustion never happens right away, which is why it's rarely addressed to the timing of falling asleep. However, the longer we remain awake in the evenings, the more mental stress we add to our lifestyle, which over time, might even lead to a burnout.

There is one more reason to go to bed early. The longer we remain awake, the higher the chance we will want to eat something. Especially if the dinner is around 6–7PM it's logical that at around 10PM the body asks for some snacks. That is a trap: whatever we eat shortly before going to bed interferes with sleep quality, as our bodies will have a hard time processing what we've eaten and digesting it while we sleep. So, instead of resting and recovering, our bodies would work part-time shifts as processing factories.

THE MONTHLY CHALLENGE: RECONNECT WITH NATURE

Quality of our energy determines the rest of our life: our mood, our relationships, our performance, and the results we get. Wouldn't you agree that the more energy we have, the easier it is to live? And the more exhausted we are, the harder it is to overcome adversity? Listening to our body, improving ourselves and following our natural rhythms can help us become more energetic, happier and, essentially, more resilient. If we optimize our lifestyle to make sure we do not waste energy, we will be able to include other exciting things and experiences that don't interfere with the training process.

Start to follow a daily schedule that is aligned with the natural rhythms. It is a simple, yet powerful strategy to tap into a new source of energy that will elevate your lifestyle and improve performance across all areas of life. By living in alignment with nature for a few weeks you can notice some (or all) of the following benefits:

- You'll need less sleep to feel recovered
- You'll feel fresher and overall happier
- You'll start to plan your day more effectively
- You'll improve your performance
- You'll feel an inflow of physical and creative energy

THE MORNING ROUTINE CHALLENGE

Unless you already rise earlier than 6AM, wake up 1 hour earlier for an entire month and spend that time exclusively on yourself. It can be getting some exercise, working on your personal projects, or just planning the day and week ahead. You can even use that time to complete the exercises in this book.

Create a morning routine for yourself, so that you know exactly what to do once you wake up. Put the simplest things in that routine and check them off as you go through it. Drink a glass of water, shower, 10 minutes of meditation and so on. Accomplishing even the smallest activity will create motivation to do more.

Increase your odds of success by adding external accountability to your challenge. Post your intent and progress on social media with hashtags #resilientathlete and #trainforadventure.

ENERGY AND VITALITY

For many athletes, exercise feels great once it is over. The sense of achievement, the rush of endorphins and of course, the physiological adaptations that make people look (and feel) strong, young, and lean. Who doesn't like that?

It does come at the price of training load and, inevitably, fatigue—both of which require energy to be conquered. Managing fatigue on a daily basis is not so straightforward. You can even think of it as a form of art. On one side, athletes need to overcome resistance (physical and mental) to improve and reach peak condition. On the other hand, that training stress is added on top of whatever is already happening in life. In a way, a resilient athlete is like a part-time tax accountant. He or she pays close attention to every nuance that affects fatigue, such as minimizing external stress factors or eating a "clean" diet, with the goal of saving as much energy as possible. They don't have the luxury to take their health for granted, and instead look for every detail to preserve it, while at the same time, gain that performance edge.

Energy is like a currency that we use to pay for our (sometimes indulgent) lifestyle. Generally, we have enough to cover most of the things we set out to achieve for the day, but then there are days when we entertain our poor lifestyle habits a little more. We stay up late, eat unhealthy food, plan more things to do than we can manage or don't give ourselves headspace to relax. All of these things put the body in high alert mode and drain precious life energy at an increased rate.

Imagine you have 100 units of energy every day. If it helps, think of it as a 100% battery charge. If you slept for only 4 hours or woke up with a hangover after going out last night, you start with 30 units less right away. You rush through the morning to get ready to work and leave on time, subtract 15 more. You're nervous about something, like an upcoming presentation, traffic, or an argument with someone, subtract 10 more units. You are constantly distracted by notifications on the phone and have to constantly refocus to complete work—another five units. That's more than half of the "body battery" gone even before lunchtime. After lunch you had a candy bar with coffee—subtract five more units due to inflammation and high alertness caused by refined sugar and caffeine. You didn't drink much water throughout the day—subtract 10 more units.

In any particular moment, it might not seem significant if we are a little under slept or a little stressed out. However, all of these extra subtractions add up and come on top of existing energy demands the body has to sustain its normal functions. So, at the end of the day we are left with just a few units to get us through the evening, let alone go for training practice.

> *Much like background apps in our phones drain the battery, unhealthy lifestyle habits reduce the energy we can use for the things that really matter.*

Our health and vitality have the power to define our life. We need energy in life to be able to realize our dreams. To learn something and grow, we need to train more and tolerate more training loads, to become more resilient. When we're low on energy, we tend to feel lazy, apathetic, unambitious, as well as more prone to skip a session, procrastinate or follow unhealthy habits. However, we can be so much more. While each of those individual stressors might account for only 1% of the total battery (or less), when we optimize a few of those we can free up a lot of extra capacity, and when there is more energy than we need, nothing feels too complicated. Imagine what you could do if you had more of it. You could lace up your shoes or hop on a bike to exercise. Play with your kids more. Start your own project. Or even volunteer and contribute more to your community.

This chapter focuses on reducing physical stress to optimize health and physiological fitness. Not focusing on pushing the body to the edge but allowing it to recover and have the capacity to improve. When we implement the core principles that create and preserve health and vitality, everything else falls into place. We look better, feel better, are more confident, and have more zest for life. As athletes, we can add more training per week, which will trigger more adaptation in the body and make us faster, stronger and more enduring.

As everyday people, we can make ourselves feel like those million dollars on a daily basis. So, take action to master your health. Create new habits that nourish your mind, body, and spirit, and access that energy and vitality to live your most unlimited life.

STRESS IS NOT ISOLATED

What actually happens when we push our bodies during training practice? For starters, in response to stress the body enters into the "fight or flight" mode and optimizes itself for performance. It releases hormones cortisol and adrenaline that raise the blood pressure and increase heart rate, as well as suppresses all non-essential functions, like digestion, growth, or reproduction. Moreover, during exercise, muscles accumulate lactic acid and hydrogen ions that gradually reduce their capacity to perform. During longer or particularly strenuous efforts, micro tears form in muscle fibers as well, creating pain. On top of all that, reserves of vitamins, minerals, water, and energy are heavily taxed. At a first glance, none of that seems to do any good for the body.

By the time we hit the shower after a training practice, our body starts recovering from the damage done during the session. Depending on how hard it has been and what an athlete does afterwards, complete recovery can take anywhere from a couple of hours to several days:

- **Energy recovery.** Ironically, this is the fastest part of the whole process. Even after a hard effort, it takes seconds for Creatine Phosphate (CP) and several minutes for Adenosine Triphosphate (ATP) to recover. This part is usually completed during the cool down when the intensity is lower.

- **Reserve replenishment.** When the body is low on resources (water, vitamins, minerals, glycogen), it doesn't operate effectively. Instead, it tries to preserve whatever is left. Carbohydrate recovery (aka glycogen replenishment), rehydration and restocking of vitamins and minerals are subject to how well an athlete nourishes him or herself after a training practice. While it can take as little as a few hours, it may also take several days because other recovery processes depend on it.

- **Waste removal.** Flushing out metabolic waste that has been accumulated during the exercise (like lactic acid and hydrogen ions) depends on the intensity of the session. It can take as little as a few hours for a short and easy effort or several days for a long and particularly strenuous one to clear.

- **Re-building muscle damage.** While protein synthesis by itself is a long process, muscle tightness and inflammation can slow down the speed at which the body delivers oxygen and nutrients to the muscle. On average, it takes 24–72 hours for muscles to recover from an intense session, but it may take as long as five full days to heal micro traumas in muscle tissue.

Training does not make an athlete fit; it's the recovery that follows what does the real magic. **Stress, either physical or mental, is only a trigger for adaptations to take place.** The final step for the body to return to a normal state, is to calm itself down. Only once all recovery processes are completed, the central nervous system can finally switch off that high alert mode and, eventually, allow the body to supercompensate and grow stronger. All of it, essentially, means that doing even a moderately hard training session several days in a row is only forcing the body to accumulate more stress and reduce the capacity to perform.

The important thing to note is that our body does not understand the difference between training stress or life stress. All it knows is that there's a threat and action has to be taken. Yes, we do not need to heal micro-tears from the intense pressure of being stuck in traffic, but the body's response is, essentially, the same. High alert mode is on, cortisol and adrenaline are released, and the body starts to burn through the reserves of energy, water, and nutrients at an increased rate. Be it mental stress from having an important presentation at work, physiological stress from catching a cold or not having slept well, or even emotional stress from looking after the kids who are being mischievous. All of it feeds into the overall stress that we experience and makes the training process a little harder than we might have initially planned.

Stress puts more load on the immune system, making it operate less efficiently and makes a person more susceptible to illnesses. White blood cells that should be fighting bacteria, are instead busy fighting cortisol. It is particularly visible in colder months of the year when the body works harder to stay warm and—as everyone around becomes sick—requires even more energy to fight bacteria and remain healthy.

In such conditions, catching a cold might be a result of just one session done too hard. Or putting the body through a little more stress than usual. In fact, a friend of mine with whom

I trained side-by-side for years, used to be very punctual in catching a cold. We followed the same training program and were in roughly similar shape. Yet, once studies began in September, he would always have high blood pressure before afternoon training practice, and every year without fail, right around late-October when the weather deteriorated, he would catch that cold.

Just like the body requires time to recover from a training session, it also needs time and space to overcome smaller stresses of life. A resilient athlete is not necessarily the fastest or the strongest one physically, but instead the one who slows down and breaks down the least. The one who is able to sustain the training load, resist illness and just keep going, whatever the odds. That momentum comes from the way that an athlete supports his or her body outside of the realm of training. Resilient athletes try to minimize non-training stress to optimize energy, and as a result, they not only recover from training quicker, but also their immune system works more effectively.

Results we get in sports are subject to how much time and effort we put into training (and maybe a little luck). However, how long we'll practice it, as well as how active and healthy we'll remain as we get older, will be determined by our lifestyle.

We recover from the stress of daily life in the same way that we do from a training session. So, why not take it beyond just the training process and make it part of our lifestyle? We can incorporate micro-recoveries into our life through simple lifestyle changes. To minimize the energy-draining effects and make sure we preserve that body battery for the things that are meaningful to us, and, as a result, be better prepared to face the inalienable adversity. The effectiveness of the recovery process (in training or as a whole) stands on three distinct pillars: reduce inflammation, mobilize, and oxygenate.

SNEAK PEEK: STRESS AS A TRAINING TOOL

I have been there myself: too busy, too tired, burned out, overtrained, and even injured on more than one occasion. And I know how a busy, stressful, or even hot day can make training practice harder than expected. Which is why I like to think of every stress response as a micro training session that has to be considered in the planning process.

The body triggers adaptation and makes itself stronger in response to any stress: not just from training. Anything that reduces the body's capacity to perform can be used as a training tool to become more resilient. In particular, exposure to heat, cold, altitude or even hunger facilitates various physiological adaptations over time, including:

- An increase in blood plasma volume, leading to better cardiovascular fitness
- Increased oxygen consumption and improved exercise economy
- Reduction in overall core temperature
- Reduction in heart rate
- Improved fat oxidation
- Improved sweat rate and sweat onset, leading to better thermoregulation

Instead of ignoring or muting the stress, I like to tweak the training process to provide the most optimal results. For example, if I have an easy session planned or do not have an opportunity to go as long as is needed, I increase the intensity by training fasted, doing it in the heat or adding a form of respiratory training (i.e., using a device that makes it harder to breathe). At the same time, if the training is hard enough, I minimize the stress by making sure I'm fully recovered, training when it's cool, and fueling well. This approach is very useful in preparation for long-distance triathlons (half-Iron and Iron distance), as very often these races take place in extreme heat (above +30°C).

My three key principles for using stress as training tool are:

1. **Add extra stress only on easy days.** Hit your key sessions in the best environment possible and fully fresh. This will allow us to tolerate more training load and, therefore, trigger bigger adaptations. Fatigue impairs performance and

> thermoregulation, so an already hard session becomes even harder, which compromises its quality.
>
> 2. **Add stress in small increments.** Don't go out for an hour-long run in the +30°C heat or a long-fasted training session right off the bat. Start building up with just 15–20-minute exposure once or twice per week. Use the stress sparingly and build gradually.
>
> 3. **Safety first.** Even though you face stress factors, protect yourself as much as possible. Wear sunscreen. Take water and a small sugary snack (like a few dates) with you just in case.

PILLAR 1: REDUCE INFLAMMATION

For a regular person, catching a cold is annoying. For an athlete who is in the middle of the season, it's exasperating to be forced to pause and have several weeks of progress erased as a result. Especially after working so hard throughout the year to get in the best physical condition. I know that because I have been there myself: in my best shape, full of ambition, yet sidelined by a virus. Not listening to the signals, thinking about why things like that always happen at the wrong times. But do they really? As frustrating as it is, catching a bug is just a small, yet very visible indicator of the stress that the body cannot handle. At any point in time, everybody carries bacteria that can cause all sorts of illnesses, yet most of the time, the body is effective at neutralizing them. That is, until it has capacity to do so in the background.

Inflammation is the body's defensive reaction to any kind of harm: from a sprained ankle or muscle damage after exercise to infection and even regular stress. **It is an emergency state during which the immune system investigates the problem before signaling the body to begin the repair process and fix the damage caused.** Molecules that are released during this time (inflammatory cytokines) activate sickness behavior and produce an antibiotic effect until the body can understand how best to treat the situation. In other words, when we cause harm by physically straining ourselves, not eating healthy, having too much stress or in general not giving the body the possibility to recover, it responds by pulling an emergency break and forcing itself to "reboot." The fever that accompanies many acute illnesses is the sign of the body trying to fight back while figuring out how to do it best. As temperature kills most bacteria, it's the natural first response against all viruses.

Athletes are no strangers to muscle pain following a strenuous or particularly long workout. In exercise science, it's called Delayed Onset Muscle Soreness (DOMS), which is an acute reaction to micro-tears that form in muscle tissue as a result of its excessive lengthening. These tears become inflamed and, besides pain, can also result in increased blood flow to the area (redness), increased body temperature (heat), and fluid accumulation (swelling). This causes stiffness of the muscle or joint, reduced range of motion and strength: all with the purpose of preventing more damage and giving the body the opportunity to clear out waste, replenish oxygen and deliver nutrients to aid in recovery. On a broader scale, that is what's happening across the body in response to any stress factor, not just micro-tears in muscle tissue.

In an ideal world, once the body has healed, the inflammation calms down and the body returns to business as usual. After all, it is supposed to be a quick response for the body to get the needed rest or prevent the disease from developing further. **However, when the body is facing consistent stress over time (i.e., high training load, a stressful job, lack of rest, intoxication, or poor quality sleep), such inflammatory responses get habituated in the body.** Emergency states of high alertness drain energy, slows down recovery, and weakens the body. Over time, it even promotes the growth of various diseases, because those inflammatory cytokines work just like antibiotics and impact not only the bad tissues, but also the good ones: healthy arteries, organs and joints.

Imagine going for a tempo run when you experience muscle soreness. Would it improve performance? Living in a state of chronic inflammation is the same as training through pain—we push the body to work harder and burn through our reserves quicker.

During training, we inflict damage on our body in an attempt to make it stronger. However, if we do not allow it to fully recover, then there's no benefit from all that hard training. The body is always injured, constantly working hard to heal itself, and never 100% ready. Instead of growing strong, it slowly destroys itself. Moreover, there is a growing body of evidence which shows that the inflammation level directly affects recovery after exercise. In particular, people with chronic inflammation are less able to increase or maintain their muscle mass in response to resistance training.[1]

Even though inflammation is part of a normal adaptation to training, we need to allow time for the body to heal and recover; otherwise we risk destroying ourselves. As athletes, we want to live a healthy lifestyle that keeps inflammation low most of the time, with some acute spikes to stimulate growth. But how can we tell whether we are suffering from chronic inflammation? After all, early symptoms—fatigue, discomfort, and pain—might go unnoticed amidst the training process.

Turns out, chronic inflammation is a trend that can be revealed during routine bloodwork. Top athletes do it on a monthly basis to make sure that they keep their levels under control. In particular, highly sensitive C-reactive protein (hsCRP) levels rise when the body is in a high inflammatory state, such as fighting an infection. Other biomarkers that will often be present are elevated creatine kinase (CK) levels, an increase in white blood cell count and the stress hormone cortisol. Of course, in such a physical environment like competitive sports, it's not possible to keep inflammation low all the time. However, having the data and confirming it against the signals the body sends helps to better determine what it is going through and decide what is best.

In particular, the following symptoms are most often attributed to high inflammation markers:

- Frequent infections or inflammation related injuries—tendinitis, bursitis, fasciitis, etc.
- Body and joint pain and/or stiffness
- Elevated heart rate
- Headaches, brain fog or lack of energy
- Chronic fatigue and insomnia
- Depression, anxiety, or mood swings
- Gastrointestinal complications: constipation, diarrhea, acid reflux, etc.

---

1   According to a 2017 research paper titled "Inflammation Relates to Resistance Training–Induced Hypertrophy in Elderly Patients" published in the journal *Medicine and Science in Sports and Exercise*.

While acute inflammation is caused by a direct stressor, chronic inflammation is usually caused by lousy lifestyle habits. Behaviors that by themselves harm the body not as much as that one single stressor, but compound into an even greater impact over time. The principle behind staying healthy throughout life is the same as staying healthy throughout the challenging season (i.e., flu season), so reduce inflammation as much as possible by scaling down the overall pressure on the body. Pay attention to the warning signals it sends (high blood pressure, elevated heart rate, fatigue, etc.) to find that balance between challenging yourself and pushing it too far. Manage training stress to ensure you fully recover on a consistent basis (see Chapter 15). Clean up and optimize your diet (see Chapter 11), and give yourself more headspace and reduce mental stress (see Chapter 12). Optimizing the lifestyle in such a way is a great way not only to become physically resilient, but also to maximize energy, get better results and live a long, vibrant life.

STRATEGY: COLD IMMERSION THERAPY

Humans have used cold for centuries to treat acute pain and injuries. In fact, its therapeutic use dates back through history all the way to 3500 B.C.[1] Even now, cold therapy is one of the most effective recovery techniques used by athletes during the training process. A short 10–15 minute ice bath helps to reduce swelling and muscle soreness, boost metabolism and activate the lymphatic system. All of which, in turn, speeds up waste (i.e., lactic acid) removal and promotes muscle recovery.

However, besides lowering acute inflammation, cold exposure also works well in combating chronic inflammation, which impacts the overall well-being of a person. Adaptation to cold has similar positive effects to that of consistent exercise. Moreover, it's a great tool to train emotional regulation, as you learn to remain calm in a stressful

---

1   *The use of cold dates back to The Edwin Smith Papyrus—the most ancient medical text known, dated 3500 B.C.*

environment when the mind is freaking out. Based on research, some of the long-term benefits to physical and mental health from consistent cold exposure include:

- Mitochondrial biogenesis (growth), which leads to more energy and better endurance
- Increased pain tolerance
- Improved thermoregulation (in both cold and warm weather)
- Improved mood and focus and as a result of dopamine and norepinephrine release into the bloodstream and brain
- Increased metabolism
- Improved fat oxidation
- Improved sleep and reduced levels of mental stress
- Improved immune function as a result of increased stock of certain white blood cells

Getting in a bath filled with cold water and floating ice cubes is not pleasant, no doubt about it. Nor should rapid cold immersion be practiced without preparation or at least medical supervision. However, it doesn't have to be that extreme: even as little as 1 minute in a cold shower is more than enough to trigger these benefits. Start with a warm shower, then gradually turn the temperature to the lowest possible and breathe deeply. Active meditation helps to control the shock response and calm the mind. As you get comfortable over time, gradually increase the amount of time you spend under cold water.

PILLAR 2: MOBILIZE

Every organ in our body is made of cells. The healthier they are, the more energy and vitality we experience. Cells require oxygen, water, nutrients and the ability to remove waste to live. Each of these four processes is equally important and when either of them becomes impaired the efficiency of cells diminishes and with that health and the quality of life declines.

Our lifestyle determines the overall load we place on the body. When that load is too high and the energy levels decrease in response to the demands of daily life, the body's functional efficiency drops. It is no longer able to deliver oxygen, water, and nutrients as efficiently and the process of waste elimination slows down. As a result, the body starts to retain more, pushing excess waste into the tissues (i.e., fat). In fact, the reason for many diseases is the accumulation of toxins which the body cannot eliminate quickly enough (or at all) because it is busy doing other things.

Our face is one of the best indicators of what is happening across the body, as it has the highest number of nervous connections. So, when we are pushing the body beyond what it is capable of, the face will show it. When there's too much waste (like toxins or lactic acid) that the body cannot utilize well, it shows up on the skin: through pimples, acne, and other abnormalities. It is one of the ways for the body to get rid of toxins it has and for a person to notice that something's off. These abnormalities are signals that there is too much stress in the body and it cannot process it well. The best strategy would be to take a day or two off to recharge, recover, understand what the body requires and get things back into balance. Instead, more often than not we use creams or medicine to push back or hide those signals.

Lymph transport is slow and sporadic, as are all garbage trucks. Compared to the blood system, the lymphatic system does not have a heart to pump it. The propulsion of the lymph comes from contraction and relaxation of adjacent muscle tissue. In other words, it is our job to drive that garbage truck around our body. Movement activates the lymphatic system, allowing waste to be removed efficiently and nutrients to flow quicker.

Movement

The lymphatic system depends primarily on muscle activity in the body for its circulation, which is why a sedentary lifestyle creates a major problem. People who move less throughout the day develop a sluggish lymph system. As a result, the body does not clear itself of waste as efficiently. If you ever experienced migraines after a day at the office, that's an example of the lymphatic system becoming overloaded due to accumulating toxins (from unhealthy snacks and coffee) and the inability to move them out quickly enough. Hangovers are another example.

For an athlete, keeping the lymph moving makes all the difference in the world. It speeds up the recovery process allowing us to include more training and, as a result, improve more. Moreover, keeping the body clean in such a way helps to maintain health and physical resilience throughout life.

Even though it might be the last thing that comes to mind after a hard effort (or an intense week), it is important to move the body to speed up the process of cleaning up metabolic waste. Even after the training is done. Lactic acid, hydrogen ions, hormones adrenaline and cortisol—all of it is carried out by the lymphatic system which needs to be activated. Which is why active recovery is more efficient than passive recovery. Very light exercise (like an easy spin on the bike or a short hike) on the day off from training is a great way to flush out those waste products from the body, promote blood flow and normalize internal processes. In fact, one of the reasons why exercise over time reduces chronic inflammation is because it stimulates lymph transport and blood flow, which doesn't allow toxins to accumulate.

Movement does not necessarily mean a structured or a particularly intense training session. Any form of exercise is a good start:

- Take the stairs instead of elevators
- Use a standing desk to work and practice having "walking" meetings
- Don't take the public transport if you need to travel less than 2 stops away
- Park the car further from the entrance to walk more
- Commute by bicycle
- Challenge yourself to walk 10,000 steps per day

Massage and Compression

Besides body movement, a great way to activate the lymphatic system is to use compression and massage. It can be done through manual techniques, inflatable or other devices (i.e., massage boots) and even clothing (socks, pants, etc.). In fact, compression socks were originally invented for travelers who sit a lot in an airplane and don't move much. At some point runners and other athletes started to use compression gear to reduce swelling and muscle soreness, increase blood and lymph flow, improve muscle oxygenation, as well as promote lactate and metabolic byproduct removal to aid performance and recovery.

Massaging has a wide range of benefits for the body, one of which is promoting lymph flow. In the same way, the body movement does, massaging the muscles, whether it is done for a whole body or one specific area, helps to reduce the pressure and speed up the recovery of tissues and cells. In particular, lymphatic drainage has become a popular form of massage due to its regenerative nature. Compared to traditional techniques, a therapist would use light pressure to move the lymph fluid through its vessels and in that way promote the detoxification of the body.

A deep tissue massage, on the other hand, has a different goal. It helps to open up tight areas that might be preventing effective blood or lymph flow, as well as increase the range of motion. Self-massage and foam rolling are two great alternatives for this.

Flexibility and Mobility

Muscle or joint tightness is another aspect that slows down the recovery process because it slows down the blood and lymph flow. Besides that, it can also create imbalance in the body and become a recipe for discomfort or injury. For example, tight or immobile hips is a frequent cause of knee pain. The pronation of the foot enables the ankle, lower and upper leg to roll inward, but if the hip joint lacks mobility, the knee is what bears all the load.

This can be prevented with a simple practice of targeted stretching and mobility exercises with the goal of returning the muscles to their original length. **Flexibility exercises focus on relieving tension through lengthening the muscle.** This reduces the tension caused by overusing the muscle, as well as helps us to recover faster (thanks to faster oxygen and nutrient transport). During mobility sessions, however, tension is relieved by moving the joints through a full range of motion and in that way, eliminating the possibility of muscles and tendons pressing on each other and the nerves (causing pain). On top of that, mobility sessions build strength in supporting muscles, allowing them to reach a greater range of motion and support natural movement patterns (see Chapter 16 for more details).

PILLAR 3: OXYGENATE

The most important component of human health is oxygen—without it the body would shut down in a matter of minutes. Once oxygen enters the blood via the lungs, it gets picked up by the hemoglobin and distributed to all of the body's trillion cells to generate adenosine triphosphate (ATP)—energy. The more oxygen we are able to take in, the more energy the body is able to generate, which is why proper breathing is paramount in order to maintain health and create an active lifestyle. When we breathe better, we feel better. Besides that, although the efficiency of the lymphatic system is dependent on the level of our activity, the movement from the act of breathing alone is like a pump that can help to facilitate the process of waste removal. In other words, efficient breathing improves the body's performance by means of oxygenating the muscles and the cells while at the same time speeding up the process of waste removal and preventing inflammation.

But what does efficient breathing mean? After all, we do not have to think of the breath—it's instinctive and happens by itself. Turns out, we have a role to play in it too. The primary muscles that control the process of inhalation and exhalation are the diaphragm, the muscles between the ribs (intercostal), and muscles in the abdomen. Take a deep breath and observe what happens to your shoulders. Do you lift them in an attempt to get more air in? If so, there's a high chance you're not utilizing the power of your diaphragm fully and instead, the effort comes from the neck muscles. These are smaller and weaker than the rest of the respiratory muscles, so should account for a smaller share of the effort used to inhale or exhale. **That is why a natural way to breathe is what they call belly breathing.**

When we look at the babies, we can see their belly expanding and collapsing on every breath—not their shoulders or chest. It happens naturally for children and look at how much energy they exude, despite having much smaller lung capacity (1.25 liters for an average 7-year-olds versus 5 liters for an average adult). They breathe deeply and instinctively, while adults tend to develop a more shallow breath. To a large extent, this happens as a result of the lack of mobility, but also because in a non-active lifestyle, humans do not need that much oxygen to survive. So, the body adjusts by limiting its capacity, which also limits the amount of energy we generate. Deep diaphragmatic breathing has an enormously positive impact on health and performance. Utilizing the lung capacity fully enhances the body's ability to carry oxygen, speeds up all cellular processes (i.e., digestion, growth, healing, detoxification, etc.), as well as lowers the load on the body in the long term. As with anything in life, we can improve the efficiency of the respiratory muscles with training.

1. To begin with, start with a simple practice of consciously breathing with your diaphragm and use the muscles in the abdomen. Focus on slow inhalation and exhalation. Breathe in through your nose, deeply pushing the stomach out and then breathe out. Ideally, the exhalation phase should last twice as long as the inhalation.

2. Try to gradually make your inhalations and exhalations longer. If in the beginning it took you 10 seconds to inhale, work to increase that to 20 seconds over time, and then even further.

3. Once comfortable, start holding your breath in between the inhalation and the exhalation phases. The most common pattern for the breathing exercise is 1–4–2, meaning that the exhalation phase should be twice as long as the inhalation phase and the holding of the breath four times longer.

If possible, do this exercise in fresh air and note that intense exhalation (until lungs are completely empty) can cause dizziness, so don't perform this while driving or doing any other activity that requires complete attention. Better yet, don't push yourself to the extremes.

CASE STUDY: THE POWER OF PRANAYAMA

Dating back as long as 5,000 years ago, Ayurvedic medicine is one of the world's oldest natural whole-body healing systems. And Pranayama is its form of resistance training for the breath. It aims to improve control over inhalation, exhalation and holding the breath through rhythmic patterns. Consistent breathing exercises that form the basis of Pranayama teach the body to utilize respiratory muscles effectively, as well as to calm down and strengthen the nervous system.

I once coached an athlete who had a very humble training experience. He was never a competitive athlete and his training totaled three 40-minute-long sessions on an elliptical machine, one 15-minute bodyweight HIIT session, and a Sunday walk with the children. Nothing spectacular, yet after I looked at the results of his VO_2max laboratory test that he sent me before our second meeting, I was astonished. At 43 years of age his measured VO_2max was 59.3 ml/min/kg, and his threshold pace was 4min/km. A regular person of his age would have a VO_2max of 30–35. A very well-trained one; maybe 50. His level was in the range of a super fit athlete in his early 20s training to qualify for the World Championships.

VO_2max is the amount of oxygen (milliliters of oxygen per kilogram of body weight in one minute or ml/kg/min) that the body consumes at maximum intensity and is often considered as a quantitative measure of endurance fitness. The more oxygen the body is able to consume at maximum intensity, the more energy it has and the longer it will take for it to fatigue.

So, how come a person with close to zero endurance training background had such a high level of endurance fitness? Turns out, he was a yogi with 10 years of experience. Besides those 40-minute-long elliptical sessions he would also make sure to do three 1.5-hour-long Yoga sessions per week and breathing practice every morning. That consistent training of respiratory muscles for many years, conditioned him to consume more oxygen with every breath and deliver it to working muscles. On top of that, consistent stretching and balance exercises that Yoga is based on allowed him to use his muscles in an effective way, resulting in a very strong starting point that takes many athletes years to achieve with "traditional" training.

THE MONTHLY CHALLENGE: OPTIMIZE YOUR ENERGY USE

Do you feel beat up at the end of the day and wake up not feeling fully rested? Has it been going on for a while? Are there any symptoms that occur every now and then (headaches, nausea, muscle cramps, etc.)? Assess the overall load you place on the body, considering the principles laid out in this chapter. Do you suffer from chronic inflammation as a result of accumulation of toxins in the body? Are you moving consistently on a daily basis (at least

10,000 steps per day) to support the lymphatic system? Are you getting enough fresh air and breathing deeply to help oxygenate the cells?

Don't look at the training process in isolation. Instead, consider the lifestyle habits that drain your energy and prevent you from recovering quickly from a training session. Ask yourself: What changes would I have to make to my lifestyle that would support me training twice per day? You don't need to train twice per day but maximizing your energy so that you can and will improve the quality of your life as a whole.

THE "ENERGIZE YOURSELF" CHALLENGE

Commit to one of the healthy habits below and repeat it **every morning** for an entire month. Each of these is a simple yet very effective practice that has the power to energize and kick-off the chain reaction that is the healthy and active lifestyle.

- 1 minute of cold shower (reduce inflammation)
- 5 minutes of deep breathing practice (oxygenate)
- 10 minutes of hatha Yoga (mobilize)

Don't be tempted to include everything all at once. Start with one and focus on making it a part of your daily routine.

Increase your odds of success by adding external accountability to your challenge. Post your intent and progress on social media with hashtags #resilientathlete and #trainforadventure

---

NOURISH FOR PERFORMANCE

There is a notion that an athlete can eat whatever he or she wants in unlimited quantities to fuel intense training. That everything that is put in the oven will burn and is good fuel, whatever the source of those calories may be. At the same time, outside the world of fitness and performance all one needs to do to stay healthy and lose fat is to cut down on carbs, switch to a gluten-free bread and replace cow milk with almond milk.

In reality, there are no two worlds out there. Foods that we eat have the same effect on everyone. If we put junk in our system, it will stress the body more than it would benefit—regardless of whether you are an athlete, an office clerk, a business owner, a nurse, or even a breastfeeding mother. Those who care about the long-term effect on health, about recovery, of course, the impact on performance, understand that it is not only about the quantity. In fact, in my experience, only a handful of individuals truly consider the quality of what they put in their bodies and to what extent the food they eat nourishes them.

This topic is close to my heart because lousy nutrition choices have been holding me back for a long time. I didn't know that you cannot out-train a bad diet, but I for sure tried my best. To me the "engine" and how hard I trained was what mattered most, so I snacked a lot, enjoyed an occasional treat (or three) and didn't care much about eating well-balanced meals, let alone veggies. A stop at a fast-food restaurant was kind of a ritual in our group after an important competition.

In fact, an entry from one of the training logs from my competitive kayaking career reads: "*Saturday, December 12, 2009: Another 30K done. Time: 2:40hr, avg heart rate 140, max 183. We were four today, each led 10min in front to keep warm (it was +1°C). Good effort but felt hungry afterwards—went to McDonalds with the group to re-fuel.*" Knowing what I know now, I would guess that I have left at least 20% of extra performance on the table. Inflammation causing illnesses and frequent colds in the off-season that forced me to skip training, the lack of energy on key workout days resulting in suboptimal adaptations, slow recovery between workouts and before important races, a lot of that could have been prevented with effective nutrition habits.

The move to endurance training presented my ineffective nutrition patterns to me on a silver platter, and gradually changed my relationship with food. Triathletes like to say that besides swimming, biking, and running, nutrition is the sport's fourth discipline. That's because during a long training session (or a race), even a little detail that at first seems insignificant can grow into a big problem that affects performance. Forgetting to add electrolytes to the drink can result in lightheadedness, loss of energy and muscle cramps. Taking in too much sugar too soon during exercise can result in gastrointestinal (GI) distress and force an athlete to seek shelter in the bushes to answer nature's call. Eating late at night can cause poor sleep and contribute to fatigue.

If a single nutritional factor has the power to impact performance in training or in a race, what about performance in day-to-day life over the course of days, weeks, months or even years? **Food that we eat has an equal power to nurture the body with nutrients or poison it with toxins.** It can energize us if the timing is right or drain the energy if we have overeaten. And just like during exercise, every small effect gets amplified over time.

As I experimented with various nutrition strategies, I became more aware of how different foods impacted my physiology (i.e., sleep, energy levels, digestion, performance, mood) and was determined to change the patterns that were not working well. Before paying attention to my diet, the quality of my training sessions varied substantially. With an updated focus, I was putting in more training volume and never felt better. My body started to operate more effectively, and the recovery became swift.

We are what we eat. **Our food patterns impact our energy and how much of it we can devote to training or other life priorities.** Saying no to a pizza will not magically make a person lean, nor do athletes eat whatever they wish to with no guilt. At least resilient ones don't. This chapter is about changing our relationship with food. It's about using it as a tool to nourish and build the body, not to cause additional damage or use it as an emotional outlet. It's about making nutrition a powerhouse and creating opportunities to generate even more energy by means of minimizing the effects of stress and fatigue.

Adopting healthy nutritional habits requires time and effort, just like physical training does. However, once in place, they have the power to elevate performance to a whole new level and, most importantly, support an athlete to sustain that for a long time. To do that,

I believe there are three core principles that help organize nutrition to support performance: nutrient density, alkalinity, and food timing.

NUTRIENT DENSITY

The reason I personally struggled with nutrition was that I approached it from the wrong side. I was looking at it from the perspective of calorie in calorie out—I eat the food and I burn it. That's it. However, during my endurance training I realized that all calories are not created equal. For instance, 700 calories at a fast-food restaurant will do little to aid in recovery, compared to 700 calories of a homemade meal cooked with high quality ingredients. Satiety from the fast-food meal only lasts for an hour, whereas that three-course homemade dinner can keep one full until the next morning.

So, what do people mean when they talk about calories in food? Well, energy, essentially. Caloric content is listed for reference on every food packaging and is used as a unit of measure to describe how much energy the body could get from a particular food. In a nutshell, this comes from the following three macronutrients:

- **Carbohydrates** (or carbs) are a primary source of energy. These are found in such foods as grains, fruits, sugars, etc.

- **Fats** are a secondary source of energy, but besides that, they also help to maintain healthy skin and regulate body temperature. These are found in such foods as oils, nuts, avocados, etc.

- **Proteins** are the body's building blocks (tissues, organs, cells) and, among other things, help to transfer molecules from one place to another. These are found in foods such as tofu, beans, etc.

At the beginning of my journey, these macronutrients were all that I focused on. I was very diligent in counting how much protein, carbs, and fats I was consuming, and even planned my meals to ensure that I was following a balanced split—roughly 60% of calories coming from carbs, 20% from fats and 20% from protein. Over the years, however, my focus in nutrition switched from **strength and size** to **recovery** and, ironically, that's what improved my fitness the most. In particular, I found the main problem with counting calories is that it is a very black and white way of thinking of nutrition.

After an intense or prolonged exercise, it's not only the energy we need to replenish. Among other things, the body also needs to normalize hormonal balance and calm down the nervous system, which requires a stock of vitamins and certain minerals. These are called micronutrients and their goal is to ensure the body functions efficiently.

Even when the body has the energy to operate, deficiency in a certain vitamin or mineral can prevent it from running efficiently. That can have a draining effect on mood, performance, energy, as well as decrease the ability to focus or even the strength of the immune system. For example, sodium deficiency prevents the body from extracting water from the gut and moving it to the working muscles, which results in decreased performance and muscle cramps. Iron deficiency, on the other hand, can cause weakness and fatigue which doesn't go away even after having a meal.

NUTRIENTS

Macronutrients
Required in relatively larger amounts

Carbohydrates
Provide energy; support digestive health and immune function

Lipids (fats)
Support cellular function and structure; regulate temperature; protect body organs; store energy in the body

Protein
Regulate cellular processes; support mechanical and structural functions; provide energy

Micronutrients
Required in relatively smaller amounts

Vitamins
Support cell function, development and growth; function as antioxidants; assist the absorption of other nutrients

Minerals
Support bone, muscular, cardiovascular and nervous system functions; produce enzymes and hormones

Phytochemicals/phytonutrients
(Not considered essential)
May help prevent chronic diseases; exert actions such as anti-inflammatory, anti-microbial and antioxidant effects

What are macro and micronutrients?

In the fitness world, there is a lot of buzz on how much calories athletes should consume to lose fat or gain muscle. However, the true value of food is not in how much energy (calories) it brings to our body, but rather how much of the important vitamins and minerals it provides. An athlete's diet should be balanced in both macro and micronutrients with a stronger focus on the latter. If we do not replenish the stock of vitamins and minerals used during the training session, the body will have a hard time relaxing. It is missing key ingredients to maintain its normal processes, which is why calorie-rich and nutrient-poor foods (like processed food or fast-food) are not aiding the recovery. Instead, the body spends extra resources to digest and process them, which further impacts performance, mood, health, and the quality of life—not to mention that we end up craving more food.

Think of your body as a car. A top of the line sports car, if you wish. If macronutrients (carbs, fat and protein) are the fuel that keeps it going, micronutrients (vitamins and minerals) are the oil without which the engine will overheat and might explode.

Every type of food has a different effect on the body because it contains more or less of certain nutrients. I like to consider nutrients to be a measure of a meal's overall quality. Those foods that contain a larger amount of vitamins and minerals per portion size are called nutrient-dense foods. **"Superfood" is the marketing term often used to describe the foods that contain the most amount of nutrients per serving.** Low nutrient density foods, on the other hand, are those that do not contain many micronutrients. Carb-rich foods in particular are often referred to as "empty calories" because while they provide energy, they often cause an insulin spike that results in food cravings and more stress on the body.

Examples of NUTRIENT-DENSE foods:	Examples of NUTRIENT-POOR foods:
• Greens: kale, spinach, broccoli, arugula • Berries (fresh or frozen): strawberries, blackberries, goji • Vegetables: asparagus, carrots, beets, avocados • Whole grains: oats, rice, whole grain pasta • Legumes: peas, beans, chickpeas, lentils • Nuts and seeds: almonds, walnuts, flaxseed, chia seeds	• Processed food: white bread, ready-made meals, fast-food • Sugary foods: cereals, sweet desserts, soft drinks • Baked and fried goods: pastries, donuts, cakes • Any alcohol

Even when the goal is to grow muscle, lose fat or become a more fat-adapted athlete, a balanced approach is key. Restricting the amount of food (i.e., dieting) or focusing too much on a specific nutrient (i.e., proteins) tips the scale and prevents the body from getting all of the nutrients required for a well-organized work. Cutting out certain foods is not the most effective strategy to achieve results, let alone remain physically resilient in the long-term. I learned that first-hand when I tried cutting carbs and eating more protein in an attempt to grow extra muscle during my intense training schedule. Five days later I found myself in a hospital with colon inflammation caused by the increased acidity of my diet.

Most initiatives to reduce carbohydrate intake or increase the amount of protein in the diet do create fast weight loss, which many athletes strive for. However, that effect is usually temporary, and the weight comes back quickly because restricting yourself is not sustainable. Nor is it fun, constantly saying no to yourself is not that inspiring. Instead, if we look for quality ingredients and consider the nutrient density of every food we consume, the body will optimize itself. That is because it strives for balance naturally. Once fully stocked on vitamins and minerals, the body can run its processes normally without craving food.

Athletes who discovered this connection have developed a new relationship with food. They focus on giving the body what it needs, not what the brain desires or marketing tells it to. They look to eat a varied diet and prioritize the quality of ingredients, because that is what helps them recover. And when an athlete can recover quickly, he or she can train more and improve, all while looking leaner and younger.

STRATEGY: STOCK UP ON FIBER

A good indicator of the quality of ingredients that go into the diet is the amount of fiber they contain. High-fiber foods typically are those that are found in their natural state (i.e., fruits, vegetables, whole grains, legumes) and most of the micronutrients in these foods are found in the peel. However, once these foods are processed (peeled, boiled, fermented, etc.) to create food products, a lot of fiber is removed and with that, a large share of micronutrients get lost.

Fiber is a type of carbohydrate that the body can't digest. Instead, it is consumed by gut bacteria—microorganisms that reside in the intestines and help to break down food and turn it into things the body can use. A diet high in fiber has many health benefits, including protection against cardiovascular disease, insulin and blood sugar stability, as well as a stronger immune system overall. On a typical western diet, a person eats 10–15 grams of fiber per day. A study backed by The World Health Organization (WHO)[1] emphasizes a minimum that is at least double of that: 25 grams. A better goal to strive for is even bigger: 30 to 50 grams.

Moreover, fiber is the body's natural way to regulate the amount of food it requires, because of the satiety effect. A person can easily drink a liter of apple juice but will probably struggle to eat nine apples which is the equivalent amount of calories. Gradually incorporating fiber-containing foods into the diet is a great way to improve the quality of it and with that, optimize the body's internal processes, speed up recovery, and improve overall health.

Going to the farmer's market and buying fresh produce has been a lead domino for myself to improve my nutrition. Having ingredients to cook from triggered a series of positive habits, like making healthy snacks and eating more greens, which brought variety into my diet and helped my body to operate better.

---

1   In reference to the study report titled "Carbohydrate quality and human health: a series of systematic reviews and meta-analyses," published on January 10, 2019, in The Lancenet.

ALKALINITY

Throughout the training process, an athlete breaks down muscle and attempts to repair the damage as fast as possible through nutrition and rest. All with the purpose of being able to train more and improve further. However, when the body suffers from chronic inflammation, it means there is something that it tries to get rid of. Something that taxes energy supplies, reduces athletic performance, slows down recovery, affects the mood and productivity, as well as negatively impacts long-term health. To a large extent, that is the result of the quality of our diet, as waste products, toxins, bacteria, and mucus that the body strives to clean originate from the foods we consume.

Besides causing inflammation, a nutrient-poor or particularly heavy diet is also acid-forming. Inflammation and acidity go hand in hand. The drop in blood pH (more acidity) comes as a result of infiltration and activation of inflammatory cells in the tissue.

To get back to a normal environment (slightly alkaline), kidneys process the amino acid glutamine that is generated by breaking down muscle tissue. The more acidic the diet, the more kidneys need to work, and the more glutamine is required to regulate the blood pH level. Ironically, high protein content of the food makes it acid-forming, which contributes to the muscle breakdown process and research shows that people who consume primarily alkaline-forming foods tend to preserve their muscle mass better.[1]

For an athlete, alkalinity of the diet is particularly important to consider, because their training process already creates an acidic environment in the body. Anaerobic exercise produces lactic acid and elevates levels of hydrogen ions (H+), both of which increase blood acidity, thereby facilitating muscle breakdown and reducing the levels of oxygen and other nutrients available for the body. Athletes can mitigate that effect by reducing the consumption of acid-forming foods, in particular: refined sugars, highly processed foods and those with high protein content (i.e., animal protein, dairy). This can help the body to operate more efficiently, recover quicker, prevent inflammation-related injuries (i.e., tendonitis), support the immune system, and with that, access extra capacity to perform.

Excessive consumption of refined sugars and simple carbohydrates (that also contain sugar) is one of the major causes of chronic inflammation. As we are enjoying the taste of that chocolate croissant, pizza or even a cold soda on a hot day, our pancreas releases the hormone insulin that helps to reduce the blood sugar and divert it to the relevant cells to be used for energy or stored as fat. Once nutrients are absorbed, insulin levels drop back to baseline. That rollercoaster of blood sugar spikes happens every time we consume something sweet and releases the stress hormone cortisol, which leads to inflammation. The higher the amount of sugar consumed, the more insulin gets released and the more stress is placed on the body.

Measuring blood glucose after a meal is a good practice to help understand how the body responds to different foods. For a healthy individual it should drop below 100 mmol/L one hour after a meal. If that is not the case, he or she needs to consult a physician and review the amount of refined sugars in the diet.

---

1   In reference to the research titled "Alkaline diets favor lean tissue mass in older adults," published on December 8, 2008, in *The American Journal of Clinical Nutrition*

Most people are not even aware that their diet is saturated with refined sugars and simple carbohydrates. They are added to almost every product we can find in supermarkets with the goal of extending shelf life. Much like unhealthy snacks, processed foods (like pre-packaged meals or fast-food) tend to be stripped of many nutrients, contain a lot of added sweeteners (white sugar, corn syrup, glucose fructose syrup, maltodextrin, etc.), high amounts of pro-inflammatory Omega 6 fatty acids and even trans fats. All of that promotes inflammation across the body and burns through the reserves of micronutrients, which slows down recovery and stimulates the development of various illnesses.

While Omega 6 fatty acids play an important role in cell metabolism, they should be balanced with Omega 3 fatty acids in a healthy ratio between 1:1 and 4:1 in favor of Omega 6. However, as a result of diets high in refined vegetable oils and foods cooked in vegetable oils (typical in a western diet) that ratio often reaches 15:1 or even 30:1. That increased share of Omega 6 in the diet triggers release of proinflammatory cytokines that—besides putting the body on high alert—promote the growth of various chronic diseases, including arthritis, diabetes, and even cancer.

Switching to a diet that is low on refined sugars brings more sustainable and even energy throughout the day, as well as reduces mood swings. However, healthy food does not taste as good when a person is used to a diet rich in sugary or processed foods. According to various studies, it takes two to four weeks to alter the gut microbiome with the bacteria that can process new types of food efficiently.

Below are a few habits that can help you get started:

- **Switch to foods that have more fiber.** Substitute wheat breads and pizza crusts for wholewheat options. Stock up on fruits, berries, and nuts. Add a smoothie to satisfy a sweet craving, especially on a warm day.

- **Substitute sugary snacks for natural options.** Simple tortilla chips with homemade guacamole. Fresh vegetables with hummus. Almond butter on a rice cake.

- **Cook at home.** Use nutrient-dense ingredients and prepare meals with lots of vegetables as a base. That will provide the flavor and all possible vitamins and minerals which the immune and nervous system will be thankful for.

- **Consume healthy fats.** Avocados, nuts, seeds (especially flax seeds high in Omega 3) and olive oil help to lower the LDL (bad) cholesterol and increase HDL (good) cholesterol.

- **Load up on antioxidants.** In response to internal and environmental stress, the body creates unstable molecules called free radicals. These are waste substances that steal electrons from other molecules and cause damage to cells. Antioxidants found in certain foods may prevent some of that damage by neutralizing free radicals. Some of these foods are blueberries, strawberries, raspberries, kale, spinach, beets, natural honey, natural maple syrup, and dark chocolate

- **Use more spices and simple dressing.** Turmeric and extra virgin olive oil (cold-pressed) have powerful anti-inflammatory effects on the body and besides being a good way to regulate blood sugar, are also great natural alternatives to anti-flu medicine.

- **Take pauses while eating to allow the body to process the food.** It takes a while for the body to send a signal to the brain that it's full, so when we eat too fast, we often end up overeating.

Another big factor contributing to the overall acidity is the consumption of foods that are harder for the body to process: animal protein, dairy, coffee, and alcohol. When these foods are ingested, the body releases enzymes that create a more acidic environment in the stomach that helps to break them down. Consuming such foods in excess and/or at every sitting puts a lot of pressure on kidneys and liver which cannot process everything in time. As a result, the food stays in the lymphatic system for longer and becomes toxic waste, promoting inflammation, slowing down important processes, and contributing to the growth of various diseases.

The lymphatic system is critical for managing the elimination of toxins from the body and when it's blocked, we become overloaded by our own waste and defenseless against attacks by viruses, fungus, and bacteria.

Feeling unwell after a meal is a sign that it is too much for the body to handle at the moment. Gas, burping, cough, headache, acid reflux, rash, vomit, low energy, and the inability to fall asleep: these are all the signals of the body trying hard to clean itself. Symptoms that are visible after eating acid-forming foods are similar to those of the body fighting toxins or allergens. Many people are not aware that they are "intolerant" of dairy products until they exclude them from the diet and find that the symptoms they have dealt with for years miraculously disappear. Next time you eat something, think of it from the perspective Will this food nourish my body or clog my lymphatic system?

In the meantime, here are a few ways to help detoxify the body:

- **Drink more water.** Our body consists of ~60% water and it's involved in virtually every process in our body. Many of the people are in a chronic state of dehydration, which makes them less efficient. Aim to drink at least 2–3 liters of pure water every day (excluding tea, juice and other liquid substances) and add some lemon to make it alkalize. Within several days, you will notice improvements in energy levels, mood, ability to focus, as well as less food cravings.

- **Consume less allergens.** Try excluding foods that commonly cause intolerances and allergies (i.e., dairy, gluten). While some people are less reactive, these food groups are harder for the body's lymphatic system to process. Regardless of whether you have an intolerance or not, minimizing extra stress on the digestive system helps to save more energy.

- **Sweat the toxins out.** The skin is one of the avenues through which the lymphatic system removes waste. Easy exercise that promotes light sweating is very effective in helping the body to recover. If you have the option, going to a sauna on a weekly basis is a great option to detoxify and support the immune system.

- **Fast for a day.** Give your body time to clean itself every few weeks. No need to push it and go on a water-only fast if you are not used to it or have a medical condition. Treat it as an offloading day instead: reduce the amount of food in half or at least exclude heavy, refined, and processed foods.

While it might look like it, eating a less acid-forming diet is not about reducing the amount of protein we get. After all, consuming a high amount of protein is important for an athlete to recover well, maintain muscle mass and perform. However, there are healthier ways to get the required amount of it than eating endless chicken breasts or downing half a dozen eggs every morning. In particular, plants contain protein in a much more balanced way that doesn't put the body under a lot of stress and drain its reserves. And while it does require combining various sources to get all the required amino acids (i.e., grains + legumes), doing so ensures that we eat a varied diet and consume a lot of micronutrients, which supports the recovery processes.

SNEAK PEEK: WHAT I LEARNED ABOUT MY BODY FROM BECOMING A VEGETARIAN

Removing meat and fish from my diet has been the single most impactful lifestyle change that I have made. I could even call it my secret weapon, even though it's not that secret. Changing my diet altered my life in all of its areas and after making the transition I felt as if I had tapped into a whole new capacity I didn't know I had.

Thanks to a quick recovery, I was able to include more training sessions, which improved my endurance and made me stronger than I was during my competitive kayaking career. It also made me leaner, maintaining a sub-10% body fat level that required no extra effort on my side thanks to a varied diet balanced in nutrients. More importantly, my energy levels, productivity and mood got to an all-time high as I combined family, intense training schedule, nine to five corporate career and launching a coaching business.

It wasn't an overnight switch, though. I used to consume a variation of animal protein at every sitting, which is typical on a Western diet. So, I made the transition gradually and experimented with no-meat Mondays and dairy-free weeks. Once I saw how well my body responded, I realized it doesn't need animal protein to perform.

It was in the middle of the training block for the New York City marathon that I finally made the switch. Everyone told me to wait until the event was over and the training stress dials down. However, my belief in the positive impact on performance was strong and, as the marathon came closer and intensity increased, I got more and more confident that a diet without animal protein is good for me. In the last 2 months, I pushed my body more than I was used to, adding extra threshold work and increasing the mileage to the point that would make me overtrained quickly. Instead, fatigue from hard or particularly long sessions that used to stay for days was all but gone within a matter of a day. Muscle soreness? Haven't felt it much ever since.

Besides reducing the inflammation and acidity, I attribute that to a more varied diet that I was forced to adopt. On a plant-based diet, there are only a few foods that provide the entire spectrum of amino acids to support muscle function. So, I had to learn new recipes and combine things like rice and lentils or beans on toast to get a "complete" protein. It was definitely more work, but worth it.

Here's a typical day of eating for me during intense training period:

- **5:30AM: Morning snack.** Avocado toast with tomatoes or a handful of dates and nuts.
- **7:30AM: Breakfast.** Granola with plant-based milk (almond, coconut), buckwheat porridge with chia seeds or overnight oats with berries.
- **10:00AM: Second breakfast.** Smoothie with spinach, banana, almond butter, hemp protein and spirulina.
- **11:30AM: Lunch.** Mixed vegetable salad with beans, nuts, and a slice of wholewheat bread.
- **1:00PM: Snack.** Homemade protein brownie or a chia pudding.
- **3:00PM: Early dinner.** Lentil dahl with rice or wholewheat spaghetti with grilled vegetables and pesto.
- **6:00PM: Dinner.** Quinoa salad with hummus and avocado or steamed vegetables with coconut oil and tofu.

FOOD TIMING

Have you ever had a training session in the middle of which your stomach felt bloated and it was troublesome to continue? Or were you in a situation when after finishing an amazing three-course meal you felt discomfort a while later? Maybe a food coma after a Christmas or Thanksgiving feast with barely enough energy to flip through the TV channels? That feeling of pressure or heaviness is a signal that the body's digestion process is slow and consumed nutrients do not reach the blood and muscles fast enough to provide energy. They drain it instead, resulting in a feeling of lethargy, fatigue or even pain.

Due to the specifics of the digestion process, our body processes various foods differently. Some require a more acidic environment (like proteins), while others need more alkaline (carbohydrates) to get broken down and absorbed into the blood. The problem is that when we consume different food groups together (and in large quantities), our body has a hard time providing a common environment to process everything efficiently. Which means none of the foods get digested quickly and they stay longer in our body, fermenting, causing bloating, gas and other discomfort. To speed up digestion and ensure all the nutrients get absorbed as fast as possible look to consume meals that consist of foods which the body processes in a similar way.

In particular, avoid eating protein-heavy foods (meat, dairy, etc.) together with starches (carbohydrates with low water content like grains, potatoes, etc.). Both of these are the heaviest food groups to process and combining them only creates a traffic jam in the stomach and the lymphatic system. Combine either of the groups with vegetables instead. The second food combining rule to remember is to avoid eating desserts or fruit after the main meal. Sugars are processed within 20–30 minutes and eating them on top of the main meal will make them ferment in the stomach, causing bloating and gas. That fermentation also causes alcohol to be produced as a byproduct which can contribute to inflammation. Desserts are best consumed as a standalone meal 20–30 minutes before or 2+ hours after the main meal.

An athlete's diet has to be focused on clean and timely eating to help replenish all that massive loss of energy, nutrients and water to support intensive training. **However, eating healthy is not only about what we eat.** ***When*** **we consume food and how we combine it is equally important to maximize the energy we have.** In fact, nutrition timing is an area where many athletes go wrong. Eating too close to the training session, not nourishing the body enough after or otherwise interfering with recovery. All of it puts additional stress on the body and prevents the athlete from living up to his potential.

> *An athlete has to consider what the body requires most at each particular time and which nutrients can provide that.*

A good practice that athletes can adopt to distribute energy evenly throughout the day and with that, improve performance, is to consume smaller but more frequent (5–6 times per day) meals. Add in a couple of healthy snack times between breakfast, lunch, and dinner to distribute the food more evenly. Salad bowls, granola, homemade energy bars are all great options and are very rich in nutrients. As none of the meals are too large, digestion happens faster and, thanks to that, recovery is quicker.

Keep in mind the following do's and don'ts of food timing to help you optimize the diet:

- **DO consider the timing of macronutrients.** Carbohydrates are most needed in the morning and before training to provide the body with quick energy. Protein, on the other hand, is required for muscle building and recovery, which typically happens in the second half of the day. Fat provides slow energy and a feeling of satiety, which is perfect before non-intensive activities. Consider also that depending on the food consumed, our bodies spend hours digesting the food before nutrients reach the muscles. Which means a heavy meal eaten before bedtime (~2 hours) will mess up the quality of sleep.

- **DON'T train hard on an empty tank.** Training while fasted is a great way to build endurance, become more fat-adapted and get leaner. However, it should be done at very low intensity—no higher than Zones 1–2 (see Chapter 14 for more details). Doing a hard training session when the body doesn't have enough energy makes it even more intense and reduces its effectiveness. It forces the body to tap into reserves and slow down its existing processes: the same effect that happens when the body is tired.

- **DO eat 2 hours before a key training session.** An interval or a long session is usually the most important training practice of the week, as it moves the performance needle the most. It also requires a quick release of energy due to a high training load. If there is not enough glucose (sugar) in the blood because an athlete hasn't eaten or the food hasn't been digested yet, the body will struggle to provide that, and the session will be ineffective. The best time for a meal to ensure nutrients are absorbed in time for the training session is approximately 2 hours. If the intensity of the session is low or the meal is not too heavy, that time can be shortened to 1 hour.

- **DON'T over-fuel during easy training.** One frequent mistake that endurance athletes make is consuming too much before or during easy sessions (in the form of sports drinks or energy/protein bars). The purpose of a long session is to build mitochondria in the muscles and teach the body to utilize fat for fuel better; this helps the body to get more efficient at low intensity. However, when we consume too much before or during the session the body continues to rely on sugar instead of fat for fuel. A good approach is to take in some sugar (a sip of sports drink or a bite of energy bar) only when hunger starts. Hunger is a signal that the blood sugar is getting low and a little nutrition helps to return it back to normal.

- **DO consume a light snack immediately after a training session.** Besides hydrating, in the first 15–30 minutes after a hard training practice, it's important to consume a small and sweet snack (like a fruit) to get some sugar into the system to activate the recovery process. This helps to replenish some muscle glycogen (stored energy) that was depleted during training and in that way reduce the load on the body. Moreover, it raises the blood sugar a little, which helps to manage food cravings that can occur after a particularly intense or prolonged session.

STRATEGY: EARLY DINNER, BIGGER BREAKFAST

Our body's metabolism is the fastest during daytime, so everything eaten when the sun is down takes more time to get properly digested. When we get full before going to bed, our bodies "stay awake" processing it, which slows down recovery. It's like having a part-time job on top of a regular job. Eating late at night is one of the major reasons why people wake up tired in the morning, need more sleep to feel fresh or generally find themselves less enthusiastic in life. Which is why one effective strategy athletes can use to radically improve their recovery is to avoid eating before bedtime.

The concept of time-restrictive eating (a form of intermittent fasting) has gained a lot of popularity recently. According to the process, a person should eat within a specific period of time (usually around 10 hours) and then let the body fast for the rest. This doesn't mean reducing the food intake, though. A person would still consume the food that he or she would normally eat, just in a shorter time window. What that extended period of fasting does is promote the secretion of the Human Growth Hormone (HGH) and reduce the inflammation. Yes, that same growth hormone that helps to build muscle, promote cell growth, slow down ageing, and do many other great things.

In a fasted and resting state, the HGH release is at its peak, which makes it the best time to recover the nervous system and heal micro-traumas caused by training. The body rebuilds itself only during complete rest and especially in the last hours of sleep (since in many cases that is when the fasting state starts). Nature has designed it so that sleep correlates with a long fasting window to make sure the body is at complete rest when it needs to recover. So, the better we sleep, the more effectively the body can build muscle and recover for the next training session.

Eating late at night shortens the window during which the body is in the most optimal state to rebuild itself and, as a result, impairs recovery. For athletes, recovery is the most important aspect of the training process, so if we are not able to recover in time for the next key training practice, then we won't be able to tolerate more training load and improve at the rate we desire. We can use the fasting mechanism to our advantage and speed up that recovery between the training sessions by extending the time between our last and first meals of the day. Not necessarily skipping dinners altogether, but rather having them very early in the day to make sure the body spends the maximum amount of time in a fasted and resting state.

THE MONTHLY CHALLENGE: DETOXIFY THE BODY

Regular people can get away with lousy eating habits and write off such side effects as brain fog, occasional headaches, joint stiffness and lack of energy, athletes are much more sensitive to that. With a lot of stress placed on the body every day we just cannot allow ourselves to lose efficiency anywhere. What we eat affects how we feel, look, perform and even how we think. And, logically, we want to ensure that food is digested properly, and we get all the good things into our system quickly.

However, sometimes we do let ourselves indulge in unhealthy foods a little more than we should. That's when we need to clean our room and re-energize. The aim of such exercise is to "reset" the diet and recalibrate it for more energy, performance, and overall good mood. We want to stop craving sugar or reaching for a snack to help unwind, and to make food work for us, not against us. The goal is not to become a full-time Tibetan monk who leads an ascetic lifestyle, but rather cut out the unhealthy part for at least a month and then add some occasional treats back (if you feel like it). As a positive side effect, this exercise can help to discover whether you tend to cover up some underlying issues (like dehydration or stress) with food.

THE "PHYSICAL DETOX" CHALLENGE

Select one of the habits below and follow it daily for an entire month. Don't be tempted to select several; take it one small step at a time.

- Drink 3L of water over a course of a day
- Exclude processed foods
- Exclude refined sugars and liquid calories
- Exclude caffeine and alcohol
- Exclude meat, fish, and dairy

Increase your odds of success by adding external accountability to your challenge. Post your intent and progress on social media with hashtags #resilientathlete and #trainforadventure

CREATE TIME FOR YOURSELF

Lack of time is a challenge that many people face, not only athletes. All of us would enjoy more hours in the day—be it for training, self-development, spending time with friends and family, or just being in nature to listen to birds singing and witness the grass growing. We are just too overwhelmed or tired to do these things sometimes, aren't we? The boss calls us just as we reach for the bag to hit the gym. The baby was crying all night and we didn't get good sleep before the interval session. There are always tons of small actions that need to be done. And just like negative emotions can stack up, over time these small demands can create an image that our schedule defines our life and there is not enough time in it for ourselves.

For most of us, the pace of life is very fast. As athletes, we tend to be overachievers and often strive to fit as much activity into our lives as possible. A regular person is probably already in a state of chronic stress from everyday life. Add a demanding training schedule on top of that and you get a recipe for burnout. Sounds absurd, yet that's exactly what many athletes do. They push themselves on every session to get a feeling of a "job well done" and pay a high price for typically marginal benefit. Over time, this practice puts an athlete into a chronically fatigued state and doesn't allow him to give 100% when it actually matters, which leads to plateaus in training, overtraining, and inevitably, injuries.

I believe many of us (regardless of age) belong to what I call the "O-Generation": Overworked, Overstressed and Overtired. Day job, business, family or relationship commitments, impact from poor diet, lack of sleep, weather—every little thing contributes to the overall level of stress and fatigue. Often to the point of burnout. Not too quickly to feel exhausted right away, though. Instead, gradually the boundaries between stress and rest become blurred and the concept of personal space gets stretched to the limit (especially with the rise of working from home policies). That's when many people find themselves in a so-called gray zone: not fully switching off to rest, but also too tired to operate at full capacity. Always pushing, but not having the energy to push hard or long enough. Never relaxing and appreciating the moment fully. Waiting for Friday in a state of chronic sleep deprivation, stress, and mental and physical fatigue, yet failing to recover over the weekend. As if living in a moderate effort—always around those 75%—and never supercompensating.

As a coach, I always consider lifestyle as a whole before creating a training program. In particular, not just how much time an athlete can carve out for exercise, but also how his or her daily life looks like and whether or not it can support intense training. It helps me understand how much load that person can tolerate at the moment, and how big of a change the training process would turn out to be. More often than not, those four-to-five hours per week that we estimate we can commit to training turn into two or three. That's because as an O generation, when we do get some "free time," we likely spend most of it doing things that don't align with our priorities (goals, values and purpose).

Doing things that are classic time-wasters—scrolling through social media, rewatching past TV series, playing video games, indulging in desserts, obsessing over the news, or endlessly surfing the Internet. The official reasons for skipping workouts are usually too much work that day, didn't have the time, not feeling well. More often than not, though, missing a workout is an attempt to give ourselves room to escape from those hundreds of minor stressors of daily life. To breathe, get some headspace, be with ourselves, even if that means using not-so-efficient coping mechanisms.

> *As human beings we have tremendous capacity to absorb pressure, stress, and turmoil. But we do not have this capacity infinitely. We need to take down time to recharge our internal batteries or we risk burning out.*

Often, athletes stop training not because they don't want to continue, but because they "don't have the time" and aren't able to integrate sport into life. The truth is that you won't "hopefully have the time" to exercise. You have to *make* that time, otherwise life will consume it with small tasks and drain your energy with tiny stressors. In this chapter, I will share with you a few effective time and stress management tactics to create that headspace for yourself and be full of energy to put in the work when it's required. To stop some of those mental background apps and free up extra capacity. To make sure you are spending your time on your terms and not someone else's.

THE EFFECT OF STRESS

Whenever we face a stressful situation, be it pronounced like being chased by a stray dog during a run or intangible like a looming work deadline, our body responds by activating the so-called "fight or flight" response. Breathing quickens, blood pressure rises and the heart beats faster, among other things. Such physiological changes are triggered by the release of the hormones, adrenaline and cortisol that prompt us to either stay and fight or flee to safety, a survival mechanism that enables people and other mammals to react quickly to life-threatening situations. Unfortunately, in the age when being attacked by a predator is possible only on a safari trip that has gone wrong, the body tends to also overreact to stressors that are not very life-threatening like traffic jams, work pressure, or even relationship difficulties.

Mental stress occurs when the area of our brain—called hypothalamus—is activated. That can happen when a person gets frightened, prepares to attack, expects a physiological impact, gets scared, angry, and so on. The hypothalamus is like a command center and communicates with the rest of the body through the autonomic nervous system that has two components: sympathetic and parasympathetic. Think of it like the gas and brake pedals in your sympathetic nervous system as it mobilizes the body and gives it energy to power through perceived dangers, while the parasympathetic nervous system activates the "rest and digest" response that calms it down after the threat has subsided. These changes happen so quickly that people are not aware of them, which is why the stress response has a lot to do with how we condition our mind. If we focus on factors that create stress, we will get more of it and vice versa.

Our focus and breathing is a great tool to guide the autonomic nervous system. When you're feeling low on energy or apathetic, use shallow and quick breaths to pump yourself up and activate the sympathetic nervous system. When you are stressed out and anxious, use slow and deep breaths to activate the parasympathetic nervous system and calm yourself down.

A stress response can be triggered in an instant, but how quickly an individual calms down and returns to normal is not fixed. It is subject to the magnitude of stress and how good a person is at regulating him or herself. Just like there is acute inflammation and chronic inflammation, there can be acute and chronic stress.

Being in a state of chronic stress is like working as a bike messenger while having a full-time job and other life commitments. Riding a bike might sound easy but spending all of your free time on it leaves the body exhausted. The same is with mental stress: feeling anxious about being stuck in traffic, worrying about something that may or may not happen or being concerned about a comment someone made about you might not sound like much, but doing it on a constant basis doesn't leave enough energy for much else in life—even being positive and happy. It keeps the gas pedal continuously pressed down, cortisol level high and body on high alert, which takes a toll.

None of the most typical symptoms of chronic stress sound like characteristics of a resilient athlete:

- Fatigue
- Difficulty staying focused
- Being easily irritated
- Sporadic energy levels (highs and lows)
- Problems falling asleep
- Buildup of fat tissue
- Low motivation, self-esteem and/or libido

STRATEGY: MEASURE STRESS USING HEART RATE VARIABILITY

Mental stress is part of everyday life and has an impact on our health, mood, energy levels and even happiness. It is an inevitable part of the lifestyle, but the magnitude of it and its impact on the training process is well within our control. The effect of cumulative stress on the body can be measured with Heart Rate Variability (HRV): the difference in the time interval between successive heart beats and a useful tool that helps to determine the body's readiness to perform.

When the autonomic nervous system is balanced, the heart receives signals from the parasympathetic system to beat slower and from sympathetic to beat faster. Which means, that when we are at rest, the heart doesn't necessarily beat consistently. It beats when the body needs more blood and the faster it reacts to these changes, the less stressed the body is. For example, if the heart rate is 60 bpm, it's not actually beating once every second. There might be 0.87 seconds between two beats, then 1.04 seconds between the next two. These variations in the timing of the heartbeat reflect the level of stress the autonomic nervous system is under. The less variation, the more stress, as the body adapts to a more consistent pattern of pumping blood. The greater the variability, the more ready the body is to perform at a high level.

HRV is a tool that can help athletes maximize the effect of their training process. It considers all factors that contribute to stress level and, as a result, impact performance: mental stress, sleep quality, nutrition, training, and even jet lag. It indicates trends in how the body adjusts to the demands of daily life and can even reveal early signs of burnout, overtraining or getting sick, so that athletes can adjust their training before they push the body over the limit. For example, if you wake up one morning and your HRV is very low and you planned a high intensity workout, you might want to reconsider and go for a recovery session or have a rest day instead. In the longer-term, using devices in such a way and HRV in particular to guide the training process helps you to become more intuitive and aware of how stress affects performance.

Heart rate variability is quite sensitive. It fluctuates throughout the day, from day to day and from one person to another, just like stress does. Which is why it is best to pay closer attention to weekly and monthly trends instead of daily measurements. Personally, I like to keep a log of my data and use a long-term average (one month) and a short-term average (7 days) to spot patterns:

- Daily measurement is visibly lower than the 7-day average = A signal to take the day easy or completely off
- The 7-day average is visibly lower than the 30-day average = A signal that the body is accumulating too much stress and needs a few days of rest or a week of easy training.

It's our response to what happens around us that activates the hypothalamus, which means the power over stress is within our control. Sure, the "fight or flight" response has a clear purpose in the face of danger, but it shouldn't be activated over every day, non-life-threatening factors like traffic, emails, bills, negative self-talk, or even personal concerns. It's not a problem if these factors are present, but rather that they occupy space in our head.

Think of a glass of water. If you hold it for a minute, it's effortless. Hold it for an hour and your arm might start to hurt. Hold it for a day and you will be exhausted. The weight of the glass doesn't change, but the longer you hold it the heavier it becomes. Concerns and worries in life are just like a glass of water: if we hold on to them a little longer, they start to hurt. Thinking about something negative for a minute is not a problem. Thinking about it for an hour might get depressing. Spending an entire day obsessing about something is exhausting and makes one incapable of focusing on something else.

The capacity to let go is directly related to the level of overall stress that the person is under. It is amplified by having little time to do all of the things we need or want to. Many people are unable to find that brake pedal just because they don't allow themselves time to "rest and digest." However, the parasympathetic system gets activated and the body starts to recover only when the threat (stress) has subsided. Living a busy lifestyle and starting every day with the thought of getting through it as quickly as possible (or waiting for the weekend) doesn't create an environment conducive to recovery. It doesn't even leave time to think about it. Much like training without fully recovering and supercompensating, living without giving yourself headspace undermines performance, drains the energy, and prevents a person from reaching the next level.

When we have limited time and mental space, we react to life because we don't have the capacity to pause and self-reflect; we jump to the next thing and then the next without rest. This is the culture of being always on and the reason why detox and meditation retreats are so popular. However, we don't need to escape to Bali to feel ourselves again. Instead, all we require is to turn inward to find that time and space. And by virtue of that, train our physical and emotional resilience.

"Spend some time alone every day."

— DALAI LAMA

Instead of focusing on external things, take the time to think of what you want and do that. Spend time without devices, news, and action points, just immersed in the moment. Ironically, what seems unproductive turns out to be the most productive time in the long term. When we take some time every day to take care of ourselves, the magic starts to happen. That uninterrupted time helps us mentally relax, figure out who we want to become, discover what makes us happy and recharge to get after it. Athletes who are able to effectively manage stress in such a way have a great foundation to stay resilient through life.

Getting more headspace and putting yourself first might sound selfish to some and laid-back to others. If you peek into social media, everyone seems to be working hard, staying up late and getting after it the moment the alarm rings. We are fed this narrative that the longer we stay awake, the more hours we can cram into the day and the richer our life will get. However, this hustle culture is booming only because it works well to attract attention and makes it easy to feel recognized for staying up later than others or having tons of small tasks to complete. No pain no gain, work hard play hard. **If we think about it, wouldn't more energy and less stress improve our performance and allow us to bring more value to others?** We could solve harder problems and achieve greater things. Honing that capacity to become your best self starts in the morning with full batteries to seize every moment.

STRATEGY: DIGITAL DETOX

Everyone has the capacity for positive transformation, and not by means of lifehacks or snake oil. True, life changes come from overcoming difficulties, but when we are in a state of chronic stress, we cannot show up at our best to face that adversity. It's like having a few extra apps in our brain running in the background and draining our focus and energy, one individual stressor at a time.

The human body was not designed to always be on, pushing through or processing something. While everyone has the capacity to overcome discomfort, that capacity has to be viewed in perspective of how much stress a person already goes through and whether he or she recovers from that. We become resilient bit by bit and we need mental recovery for that just as much as we need physical one.

Take a rest day for your brain once a week. Challenge yourself to switch off for a full day. Forget about your phone or TV and just immerse yourself in the moment. Meet with friends, learn, read, exercise, cook something you never tried before, or go for a hike and appreciate nature. Slowing down the pace gives the person headspace to think differently and put worries or concerns into context. It allows the system to reboot and bounce back stronger. Stress plus rest equals progress.

THE ROLE OF SLEEP

Sleep is the athlete's most powerful recovery tool because it's the only time when the body is in the state of complete rest. All regeneration processes take place quicker during sleep because changes in the body's physiology foster that. Heart rate slows down, blood pressure and body temperature drop, blood vessels across the body widen, helping to release muscle tension. When asleep, the body is usually horizontal and muscle activity is minimal (no need to maintain balance), which makes it easier to flush out waste products and deliver nutrients to rebuild tissue damage. Moreover, brain activity slows down, allowing the nervous system to relax and leading to improved reflexes, better coordination, stronger focus, and of course, more willpower.

Sleep is one of the most effective and tangible ways to give yourself headspace and take control of stress.

As much as sleep is essential to good health and high performance, consistent lack of it has exactly the opposite effect. Those who continuously "survive" on 5–6 hours of sleep every night may over time even feel like a different person. They may experience a grumpy mood, lack of energy, trouble concentrating or remembering things, slow reaction time or general sluggishness, lower pain threshold and less willpower. Not to mention the reduced exercise capacity and premature ageing.

Here are some other eye-opening statistics:

- A single night of sleep restriction to less than 4 hours decreases maximum aerobic performance by at least 4–7% on the following day.[1]

- One week of sleep restriction to 5 hours per night reduces the daytime testosterone level of healthy men by 10–15%[2] (to an equivalent of a person that is 10 years older).

- A typical sleep duration of 4 hours per night reduces cognitive ability (i.e., reasoning, problem solving, communication) in an equivalent of ageing at least 8 years.[3]

- On Mondays following spring daylight saving (associated with a "loss" of 1 hour of sleep) hospitals report a 24% increase in heart attack counts.[4]

---

1   In reference to the 2017 research titled "One night of sleep restriction following heavy exercise impairs 3km cycling time-trial performance in the morning" published in *Applied Physiology, Nutrition, and Metabolism*

2   In reference to the 2011 research titled "Effect of 1 Week of Sleep Restriction on Testosterone Levels in Young Healthy Men" published in *JAMA*

3   In reference to the 2018 research titled "Dissociable effects of self-reported daily sleep duration on high-level cognitive abilities" published in *Sleep*

4   In reference to the 2014 research titled "Daylight savings time and myocardial infarction" published in *Open Heart*

According to the data from the Center for Disease Control and Prevention (2014), 30–45% of people in the US are getting less than 7 hours of sleep every night. Moreover, the majority of chronic conditions (i.e., heart attack, coronary heart disease, asthma, arthritis, depression, diabetes) are more prevalent in these people compared to those who sleep more than 7 hours. Due to the high physiological demands that athletes place on their bodies, the effects of insufficient or low-quality sleep are amplified for them. Combined stress of daily life, intense training process and competitions drain energy, impair the body's ability to regenerate, and lead to accumulation of fatigue, performance drop, plateaus or even overtraining.

Instead, start tracking how well you sleep, and you will begin noticing patterns. Things like interruptions, tossing and turning (due to discomfort, stress or even a large meal) and movements are all signs of low quality of sleep. Minimizing those helps the body to relax, which significantly improves the quality of sleep and provides more energy.

Below are a few more strategies to improve sleep:

- **Sleep more.** While there is no magic number on how much sleep every individual needs for optimal health, multiple studies confirm that repeatedly restricting sleep to less than 7 hours per night causes significant cognitive dysfunction comparable to those observed after severe sleep deprivation (i.e., less than 4 hours). Athletes, on the other hand, might need 9 or even 10 hours of sleep to tolerate training and daily stress to ensure timely recovery for the next session or competition. If the schedule requires an early wakeup, add an extra nap during the day.

- **Have a set schedule.** The best way to ensure that you are getting enough sleep every night is to have a set schedule. Going to sleep at the same time gets the body used to a consistent rhythm (see the effect of circadian rhythms in Chapter 9). A sign of a good sleep schedule is when you feel rested in the morning, able to wake up without an alarm and don't need to catch up on sleep during the weekend.

- **Relax before bed.** It takes some time for our brain to switch off and start relaxing. Doing something mentally engaging (working, studying, flipping through social media) right before bed engages it even more. Instead, develop a "wind-down" routine to calm the mind before bed. It can include reading a real book (not an iPad or a phone), stretching, meditation, or very light yoga. Don't (over)eat before going to bed; it's best to go to bed a little hungry than full.

- **Invest in a good mattress and get quality bed sheets.** Too soft, too hard or an uneven surface forces the body to toss and turn searching for a comfortable spot. Qualitative bed sheets provide a soft environment for the body, allowing it to relax better and reach a more restorative sleep phase. Expensive linen is not only for aesthetic purposes.

- **Sleep in a dark, quiet and cool room.** Darkness promotes the production of melatonin. A quiet environment allows the brain activity to slow down. A cool room helps the body to regulate its core temperature. All three combined provide a good environment for restorative sleep.

THE POWER OF EFFECTIVE TIME MANAGEMENT

'You're so lucky that you have the time to train that much and stay fit. I could never do that, I'm always so busy.' That's a common response I get when talking about my lifestyle (before I share my *actual* training hours). As if I have all this free time that I can spend exercising or following my passion, because I've got nothing "important" to do in my life. However, when people learn what it takes to integrate training into a busy lifestyle, how I bend my calendar to squeeze out any "extra time" and how even a short session can be ultra-effective, their perspective changes. We don't get time for something in life—we have to create it for what's important to us. Everyone gets the same 24 hours every day, but not everyone integrates exercise and other health-improving habits in those.

I found the inspiration for this mindset shift in athletes who train for the Ironman triathlon, that grueling full-day endurance event. I am not inspired among professionals who devote 30+ hours to training and go on to set world records, but among individuals who pursue it as a hobby. An uber-productive CEO who runs a business yet finds 10+ hours to train and qualify for the World Championship in Hawaii, or A mother of three who works as a nurse and wakes up before the morning shift to get the training in. Thousands more who perform at the highest level and combine extensive training with family, a day job, running a business, traveling and many more factors that others use as excuses.

We can find time to do anything, as long as we attach a priority to it.

Sure, it's easier to exercise consistently when you are younger, have less responsibilities and enjoy a lot of flexibility. With the addition of a day job and a family, however, the structure that most athletes have enjoyed during their early years typically starts to fade away. In fact, transitioning to "adult life" is what most college athletes struggle with—they drop their training altogether only to find years later that something is missing in life. This is where time management comes into play: using the hours available as effectively as possible and optimizing life to create even more time and space to invest in yourself. For training, practicing a hobby, learning a new language, or simply being more present with family and friends.

One of the core principles of economics is the so-called opportunity cost. Meaning, the potential benefits an individual (or business) misses out on when choosing one alternative over another. We use time in the same way we use any other resource (i.e., money, energy): if we spend it on a certain activity, we have to give up the alternative that we could have engaged in. Often a person who says he or she doesn't have enough time for something goes and binge watches a new TV series, plays video games for hours, or spends time aimlessly surfing through social media. In such cases, the opportunity cost is that missed exercise that a person could have done.

It's not a lack of time, but rather a choice made in favor of "unhealthy" activities or habits, and while there's usually a block of time everyone can devote to exercise, a resilient athlete goes further and carves out more by searching for that opportunity cost within his or her lifestyle. They search for those moments spent relentlessly checking the phone, email, news, social media or engaging in any other technology addictions. They find the monotonous activities that can be combined with productive ones., and the non-important, non-urgent tasks that keep a person busy and can be either optimized or dropped. By the end of the day, these moments, activities, and tasks often add up to hours and never leave time for running, preparing a healthy meal, or even being present in a conversation.

The good news is that we don't need to give up on our athletic goals to feel energized and lead a fulfilling life. Nor on our personal ones to be a competitive athlete. With some practical changes, it is possible to combine busy life even with something as time intensive as training for the Ironman triathlon.

Training doesn't have to consume all of your free time. For amateur athletes in particular, it has to be enjoyable and complement the lifestyle instead of becoming a daunting task they have to do before they are able to relax. The secret to integrating training into the lifestyle is to make it convenient and exciting.

Here are the top five time-management tips I use to coach my athletes:

1. Count time, not distance
2. Break the sessions down
3. Have a shopping list of standard sessions
4. Use the calendar
5. Train in the morning

1. Count Time, Not Distance

A great way to manage your training time is to measure sessions in duration instead of distance. In other words, count how much you have trained in minutes and hours, not how many kilometers/miles you have covered. For instance, instead of going for a 5K run, go for 30 minutes. Or do 20 minutes of core exercises rather than chase three sets of 10 exercises. Doing so provides more certainty on how long each session will take and makes an athlete less attached to the outcome (i.e., running harder than planned only to cover the distance faster). Besides that, it also fits perfectly with the heart rate training approach where an athlete needs to maximize the time spent in a certain heart rate zone (see Chapter 14 for more).

The beauty of this method is that the time period is fixed. While estimates of how long it will take to cover the distance (or complete exercises in the gym) can easily be off, an hour-long run takes exactly that much: one hour. No rain, headwind, feeling tired, meeting someone along the way or taking too much rest between repeats will prolong that and such a session will not spill over into the rest of the schedule. Changing focus from distance and pace to overall time also helps to detach yourself from chasing a certain pace or a distance goal and paying attention to the present moment. How are you feeling, where's your mind at and how good is your form? Most importantly, enjoy the process.

2. Break the Sessions Down

Sessions that are long or include moderate to high intensity (i.e., efforts at Zone 3 and above) provide a lot of training benefits, but also come at a high cost. They add a lot of fatigue and often require several days of easy training (or rest) to recover from. Not to mention that it often takes a lot of time to get yourself mentally ready for a 2-hour-long session or one that includes threshold repeats. A much more effective approach is to shorten these sessions and do more of them instead.

Our body responds best to consistent stimulation, so try to do a form of exercise every day and avoid days of complete inactivity. Mitochondria in the cells that power aerobic efforts grow within 24 hours after the exercise but are very sensitive to fatigue. Exhaustion overloads them and limits progress, which is why having less taxing sessions means the body can recover and super-compensate quicker. Many good training sessions stacked one after the other in a training block provide better and more consistent adaptations than a very long or really hard one every couple of days.

> *The purpose of the rest period during interval training is to allow the body to recover and tolerate more time at high intensity. In the same way, having more frequent but shorter sessions allows us to increase the overall training time and, as a result, improve more.*

Breaking sessions down gives an athlete more flexibility when to execute them. In particular, he or she can make use of lunch and other breaks to squeeze in a short run, an explosive strength session, a core routine or even a Yoga sequence. If you can get at least two 30-minute lunch break workouts per week, that's an hour of training without much sacrifice. In fact, often carving out a block of time (i.e., 1–2 hours) for a longer session is not possible due to family commitments, work projects or other things. So, split it into two smaller ones throughout the day. It's easier to find 30 minutes in the schedule than a full hour, and even if you end up doing only one of those sessions, six days of 30 minutes still equals a solid 3 hours of training per week.

3. Have a "Shopping List" of Standard Sessions

For many athletes, deciding what to do in a training session is a big timewaster, especially when scheduling sessions on short notice. To avoid such a debilitating thought process, create a list of your favorite go-to training sessions and then categorize them for every purpose (endurance, strength, power, etc.) and duration (i.e., 20–40–60 minutes). So, when something changes in your agenda (i.e., meetings get cancelled, appointments get postponed) or you just have free time, no need to think about what to do—just pick the appropriate session from the "shopping list" and execute. For instance, if a meeting with friends gets postponed by an hour it's a great opportunity to do a 40-minute interval session or a 30-minute core routine. It's a much better use of time than aimlessly browsing the phone or answering emails.

If you don't have one yet, you can also create a standard weekly plan: sort of a "perfect week" example of what sessions you should complete each week. On some weeks, you will manage to stick to that plan 100%, while on others you will have to make changes (especially when traveling). It's OK to change the timing of sessions based on your personal schedule or how recovery is progressing (i.e., swap a tempo session for an easy run). Aim to get the key ones in when you are most fresh.

4. Use the Calendar

We all have free time for exercise, but we either waste a lot of it, or don't put a priority on training…or both. The best way to ensure that training sessions get completed even on busy days is to put them in your calendar, just like any work or personal appointment. Doing so attaches a priority to a training session and reserves time to actually complete it.

Start by drawing a weekly plan and schedule all important activities, things you can't or won't move, like family time, work, commute, mealtime, etc., in their respective times. It really helps to do it physically with a pencil or in a spreadsheet. The patterns we follow on a daily basis are usually known to us: we eat breakfast and leave for work at around the same time, the commute time is typically constant and even the trip to the supermarket is a routine task. For the activities where you are not sure about the time requirement (family time, dinner, meeting friends, etc.), block the amount of time it typically takes. The main idea is to become aware of your current lifestyle habits.

Once you have a core schedule with important things, you will already get an idea of how much time you can devote to exercise but go one step further. Look at the next couple of weeks and put in all extra appointments, travel or "life commitments": dentist, date nights, shopping, kids' soccer practice, etc. This is the point when you'll start seeing overlaps between your important things, appointments, and potential workouts: try to re-plan and move as much as possible to create a schedule that supports training, allows sufficient recovery, and is comfortable for you.

This is the time to get creative and think of interesting ways to incorporate training. Cut lunch from one hour to 30 minutes and squeeze in an interval session. Wake up before kids/wife to get your long workout in. Do an indoor training session in front of a TV to catch up with the series that you are watching. It doesn't have to be the same time every day but do block the time in your calendar for that.

"What gets scheduled gets done."

— MICHAEL HYATT

You can find time to do everything you need to or want to, but don't make excuses. How much time can you find for yourself if you optimize your life? Use your smartphone for productivity, not clickbait. Turn off meaningless notifications, have alarms set for important reminders. Combine training with something productive: listen to that self-development book or a podcast you have put on hold for weeks. At 30 minutes per day, a typical book can be finished within 2 weeks. That's 100 books a year.

5. Train in the Morning

If your day is completely packed with family, kids, work, travel, and other commitments, I understand. Everyone has to work; nobody enjoys losing sleep, and it's not like we can live in a cave and avoid social contact. If you are in a situation where you can't control your schedule, you will have to maximize the morning. Schedule your training and personal projects early—before the rest of the world wakes up. The later in the day you leave it for, the greater the chance for something to come up and interfere with your plans.

For most people, this is a big change and will take some getting used to. Waking up early requires changing the evening routine to go to sleep earlier. However, once accustomed to it, you might see that the energy levels and willpower are also stronger in the morning. Training early in the morning is by far the most effective time management strategy that athletes use: an hour-long training session before work on every weekday equals to 5 hours of training per week, not including the weekend. If such sessions aren't too taxing (see point 2 about breaking sessions down), an athlete can add a second workout in the afternoon if he or she wants to. More importantly, getting the training out of the way first thing in the morning clears the head for the rest of the day and allows you to be fully present: for work, family, or other commitments.

THE MONTHLY CHALLENGE: AUDIT YOUR WEEK

Every one of us has more than enough time during the week to fit in a training schedule worthy of a competitive athlete. Yes, it is possible to be in great shape with as little as 5 hours of training per week. In fact, with an effective program, that can be all you need to finish in the top 10% of any major competition, if not faster. All it takes is less than an hour per day.

Think of it like this: out of 168 hours we have every week, 5 hours is less than 3 percent of our available time. Even if we reserve 8 hours for work on weekdays and 8 hours for sleep each day, there are still 72 hours left in the bank. That is more than enough to include training without sacrificing the rest of life. This challenge will help you discover just how much extra time you can have each day to do what's important to you: be it training, developing healthy habits, getting quality sleep, meditating or other life priorities.

THE SCHEDULING CHALLENGE

Step 1. Put your week into a spreadsheet and record each activity that you do by hour. Don't be tempted to skip big blocks and put something like [*9*AM *to 5*PM—*at work*]. Instead, be diligent and log in every detail and every distraction, as if it were your taxes. How long does it take to get ready in the morning? How often do you check your phone? How many minutes do you spend aimlessly browsing the news sites or flipping through TV channels? How much time do you spend getting down to the smallest detail in every email you receive? You might notice many meaningless tasks and distractions you engage in without noticing. Those minutes and hours add up to days of wasted time.

Step 2. After auditing your schedule, create a new spreadsheet and draft your ideal week. Put in your family, training, meal-time, work, rest, and other appointments. Put in healthy practices you want to implement, like meditation, morning yoga, journaling or even cooking healthy meals. Once your days are all scheduled out, follow the plan for a week. Review how well you did and adjust where necessary.

Increase your odds of success by adding external accountability to your challenge. Post your intent and progress on social media with hashtags #resilientathlete and #trainforadventure.

PART III

Training

TRAIN FOR ADVENTURE

Have you ever been in a situation where you have shown up, done all the work, went what you thought was the extra mile only to find yourself exactly where you were before, making little to no progress? I know how frustrating it feels, because a year after making my first national team that was exactly where I found myself—struggling to improve further. I was getting out there, often three times per day, training more than I ever did, doing all the intervals as hard as possible, yet the progress was very marginal. At the end of the season during the VO_2max testing in a laboratory all the parameters—maximum oxygen uptake, time to fatigue, aerobic and anaerobic thresholds—remained on the same level as they were in March. Which meant that my fitness level had not improved throughout the season despite the intense training schedule.

Somehow, the method that got me to the national team had stopped working. It felt as if I hit a ceiling and training more was not helping. Not that I could physically add more to my schedule—I was constantly tired already. So, I asked the expert at the lab what I was doing wrong and once she saw my training schedule, she was surprised I haven't yet been to the World Championships—the workload was right on point. She helped me understand that the time I put into training is not directly related to how much I improve. It has to be a quality effort if I want to see sustainable results and with my disorganized approach of more and harder, I was just scraping the surface. Yes, it worked so far, but only because I had put in a lot of volume.

As if I used a hammer to tighten the screws; it can do the job but requires a lot of effort and is not very efficient. To grow further, I had to slow down and focus on the quality of every training session with the purpose of triggering timely and targeted adaptations instead of getting stuck in the eat-sleep-train-repeat limbo. It meant adding more variety, developing different speeds, becoming more focused in strength training, and adding a mixture of activities that together turned me into a more well-rounded athlete. Remember Mark from Chapter 2 who was struggling to get better at swimming? I was slowly becoming conscious of my incompetence and had a lot of deliberate practice ahead of me.

Spending an entire season to achieve minimum progress motivated me to reset and look at my training from a holistic perspective. That autumn, I focused on putting the pieces in the correct order as per the feedback on my VO$_2$max test results. The next spring, my aerobic threshold had already grown higher thanks by and large to the focused low intensity cross-training I did over the past 6 months. That was while limiting training to one session per day. If I was able to find extra performance on less training, how much can a regular person improve or reduce fatigue if he or she focuses on quality? Throughout my coaching career I found the same pattern among many athletes—they burn themselves out in an attempt to squeeze in more training and get faster. Sometimes these attempts are inspired by what World-class athletes or other influencers share on social media, but most of those efforts are not focused and are often harder than they should be. In a way, many athletes see themselves building a Ferrari engine, but trying to put it in a VW Golf body and expecting it to handle well. However, that kind of structure is not designed for a high performance and will deteriorate and break down eventually (i.e., injury, overtraining or even illness).

> *If getting better at any sport was only about training more and harder there would be more happy, strong, and fast athletes.*

Physical fitness directly impacts our overall well-being. Being strong, fast, flexible, and agile is required not only to complete a marathon, but also to have a better quality of life. You'll be able to run after your kids, build a house, not to mention to enjoy all those crazy adventures we dream of, like going to the surf camp, trekking in the Himalayas, or kayaking among the Fjords. This is why fitness shouldn't come at the expense of health.

Athletes don't have to lose the passion to run after going through the process of training for a marathon or smash themselves in any other way to get good results. Nor do they have to put their entire lives on hold and focus on one goal or one race for months and years. Life doesn't work that way. **Becoming the best version of yourself is about approaching it like**

a professional athlete, through variety and balance. That means asking yourself, '*What are the steps that I need to take to put myself in the best position for success across all areas of life?*'

At this point in the book, you are well on your way to becoming a resilient athlete. There is purpose and direction thanks to the mindset practices you have learned and applied in Part I, which makes showing up easier. And there's energy and momentum thanks to the lifestyle habit change you practiced in Part II, which helps the body to recover faster and tolerate more. The chapters ahead will give you the strategies you need to make the training super-efficient and support your adventures without keeping you drained and exhausted. Think of it as training for adventure, not performance.

A WELL-ROUNDED ATHLETE

Too many highly motivated athletes are driven by accumulating training hours and, as a result, lose sight of the big picture of performance evolution. Often in the quest for personal glory, such athletes rely on high intensity training to trigger growth because it produces quick and visible results (i.e., speed or muscle gain). In reality, such isolation puts a limit on long-term progress and can contribute to plateaus, frustration and burnout. The truth is, those very intense and impressive workouts that we see from World-class athletes, influencers or even our friends, are just the highlights and represent a small part of a balanced training process. Typically, less than 10–20% of the total volume. Imitating that can add unnecessary fatigue and disrupt the gradual progression of the training process.

When we focus too much on one area, some other part of our life does not get the required attention and becomes the bottleneck. For example, a person's relationships with family members can suffer if he or she spends all their time and attention on work topics. As a result, that person will experience more stress and won't be able to show up at 100%. The same principle applies in training. Consider Anthony who is a middle-aged man who recently took up running to stay in shape and unwind after a day in the office. He works a nine-to-five job at a management consulting firm and spends a lot of time at the desk reviewing income statements, drafting process blueprints, and creating slides for the owners of the companies he advises.

The prolonged time that Anthony spends sitting is reflected in his poor posture, tightness in the joints and limited range of motion. His shoulders are hunched forward as a result of tight chest muscles, which reduces his breathing capacity. His hamstrings and glutes are tight and weak because they are not used while sitting, which shortens his running stride and makes it less powerful. So, when Anthony runs, the body cannot operate at full capacity; it compensates for the lack of mobility by spreading the load on less efficient muscle groups, and as a result, becomes tired faster. That is Anthony's bottleneck: while high intensity training will trigger some adaptations, in the longer-term, muscle tightness will prevent him from substantially improving his fitness. Instead, it will only contribute to muscle imbalance and, most probably, will result in pain or injury.

In a way, most professional and elite athletes do have a secret. That is the knowledge and experience they have gained over years of training and racing which helps them to tailor the training process for their individual needs and maximize the effect. More importantly, they have built strength and stability in supportive muscles and joints over the years of consistent, easy training, which allows them to utilize their body's full capacity and process more training stress. **It is this foundation that separates top athletes from the rest, not necessarily hard intervals or more hours.** Athletes who are just starting out generally don't have that background and they are much less resistant to fatigue due to limited range of motion, lack of core strength or less developed aerobic capacity. The "secret" is, therefore, to focus on foundation and becoming a well-rounded athlete, *not* on adding more intensity.

A resilient athlete is capable of performing across a variety of sports, activities and tasks. He or she can embark on a multi-day cycling adventure, join friends on a ski holiday, travel to a distant place to spend time in a surf camp or even summit a mountain. Being confident in one's own abilities provides a lot of freedom to have more profound experiences and enrich your quality of life.

That well-roundedness comes from a mix of three factors:

- Aerobic fitness
- Functional strength
- Skills and conditioning

All of these factors should work in tandem to allow the athlete to utilize his or her full capacity. On its own, being physically strong or able to run fast is just a single piece of the puzzle and provides limited benefits. For example, if a person focuses exclusively on building endurance (through running, cycling, etc.), he or she might struggle with activities that demand strength (i.e., carrying a heavy backpack or ascending steep routes during long trekking days). On the other hand, if a person is strong and enduring, but struggles with balance and isn't comfortable in the water, he or she will struggle to learn to surf and enjoy the process of catching a wave.

Having such a holistic perspective in mind is a driver to retain a more balanced approach to training and performance. By shifting the emphasis away from simply training and placing equal importance on each of the three areas, athletes can make intelligent decisions throughout their performance journey and retain a strong purpose behind the entire process. It also ensures that each of these essentials is a part of the comprehensive plan and not merely an afterthought.

Aerobic Fitness

Through years of consistent training, athletes develop many characteristics that support their high-performance lifestyle. Base strength, optimal technique, agility, flexibility, coordination and even racing experience, among other things. However, one specific factor that allows them to endure more, recover quicker and, essentially, maintain their fitness throughout their life is aerobic capacity. This factor is how effectively the body can utilize oxygen to produce energy.

A molecule called ATP (adenosine triphosphate) is the "'energy currency" of the body. It powers most cellular processes that require energy, including muscle contraction required for sport performance. Consider a hypothetical situation when a person is trying to escape the claws of a grizzly bear. That person who was unfortunate enough to face the bear will most likely blast off the scene and run all out for 5 to 10 seconds. After that, he or she will slow down, maybe look around, but will continue running pretty hard for a few minutes until breathing becomes difficult and muscles start getting heavy and aching.

That's when a person will have to slow down further or even switch to a walk to carry on moving. Even despite expending a lot of energy in the beginning, he or she will be able to continue walking for hours. These three stages reflect three different energy systems that operate in the body:

- Intense efforts of 6–10 seconds are powered primarily by creatine phosphate (CP) and ATP stored in the muscles. This system is known as **the ATP/CP system** or alactic system, because lactate is not produced as a byproduct.

- Once the body has exhausted the supply of CP, it moves to **the lactate system** during which the glycogen (carbohydrates) stored in muscle tissue and liver is broken down into glucose and used to generate ATP. Hydrogen ions (H+) and pyruvate are created as byproducts and in the absence of oxygen pyruvate turns into lactate.

- As the length of the effort increases (typically over 5 minutes) and intensity decreases, **the aerobic system** becomes more dominant. In the presence of oxygen, the body uses carbohydrates, fats, or proteins to produce ATP.

A person who is more trained and has a better aerobic capacity will be able to run faster for longer after those initial few minutes of very intense running, whereas an untrained person might even need to stop to recover. The word **aerobic** means that the body utilizes oxygen to burn macronutrients and generate energy in mitochondria. In prolonged activities when intensity is low to moderate, the body will use fat as the main energy source and preserve valuable glycogen (stored carbohydrates), so that it's available in case exercise intensity increases and the body will need to produce energy quicker. Out of all three, aerobic is the most efficient energy system and provides the most energy. Even though it's the slowest, it doesn't mean it's reserved for walking pace; elite runners can maintain a 4:00 min/km (~6:30min/mi) pace for hours, whereas for most it's manageable for a few minutes only.

The ability to operate aerobically and burn fat for fuel is a key factor for athletes. The body can only store around 1,500 to 2,000 calories as glycogen (in muscles and liver) that can be used for quick energy. That is enough for around 1–2 hours of intense exercise and when the body starts to run out of glycogen performance plummets—a person starts to feel tired, lose power, get dizzy or light-headed, become disoriented and unable to maintain any form of momentum. That is what marathoners refer to as **hitting the wall.** On the contrary, even the skinniest person will have ~70,000 calories of fat that he or she can use to operate for days. And if we can train the body to rely more on its aerobic energy system, we can tap into those fat stores and use less glycogen—**meaning we can maintain the speed or intensity for longer.**

	AEROBIC (long-term)	ANAEROBIC LACTIC (short-term)	ANAEROBIC ALACTIC (immediate)
Fuel source	Macronutrients (carbohydrates, fats, protein)	Glycogen (stored carbohydrates)	Stored ATP and CP (creatine phosphate)
Limiting factors	Body's ability to process oxygen	Production of H+ ions and lactate limit capacity to 10 seconds to 3 minutes at maximu m intensity	Reserves of ATP and CP limit capacity to up to 10 seconds
Intensity of exercise when system is dominant	Low to moderate (to a lesser extent during high intensity)	High to very high	Explosive
Abilities developed throughout the training process	*Aerobic power:* Resistance that the body can overcome while utilizing oxygen *Aerobic capacity:* The ability of the body to supply muscles with oxygen	*Muscular endurance:* Ability of the muscles to resist fatigue when performing at high intensity *Power:* Moving against resistance as fast as possible	*Speed and explosiveness:* Ability to produce maximum force or develop maximum speed (up to 10 seconds)

Overview of energy systems and their usage during exercise.

There is a misconception that aerobic training is not beneficial for high intensity sports and short races (i.e., 100-meter sprints). However, with the exception of a few athletic events, no sport is purely aerobic or anaerobic. Even high-intensity activities such as surfing, BMX, rock climbing or even boxing that include lots of jumps and short bursts are predominantly aerobic thanks to periods of rest: in between waves, tricks, explosive moves or boxing rounds.

During that time the heart rate is elevated, and the aerobic system has to be strong and robust to allow the body to recover quickly before the next intense effort. On the other hand, in such long events as the marathon or long-distance triathlon besides relying on the aerobic system to power the movement, the body also uses glycogen and stored ATP/CP in such high-intensity situations as race start, powering over the hills, surging to overtake someone and so on.

Any form of exercise uses all three energy systems, but in different proportions. The longer the effort the more dominant the aerobic system is, but even though an athlete might be burning primarily fat, a steady supply of carbohydrates is still required to break it down into an energy source. Intensity of the exercise determines the predominant system and thus the effect it will have on the body.

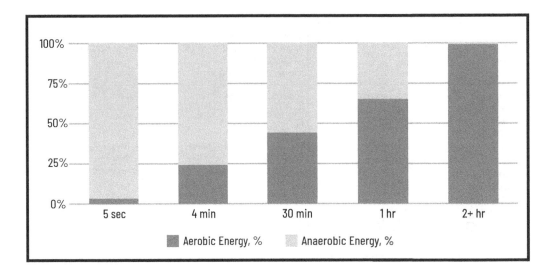

Approximate relative contributions of aerobic and anaerobic energy for varying durations (assuming maximal maintainable intensity)[1].

The majority of athletes can benefit from focused aerobic training because improving their aerobic capacity will make an athlete faster and more efficient in everything he or she does, be it training for a race, going on a hike (single- or multi-day) or even playing with children. While high-intensity (anaerobic) training may increase speed and muscular endurance, training aerobically creates a strong base for an athlete to do so. Think of the training process as building a house. The bigger the house the deeper and more solid the foundation has to be. You wouldn't start putting the roof and the windows (high intensity speed intervals) until the base and the walls are in place (aerobic fitness).

---

1   In reference to a study titled "Energy Systems: A New Look at Aerobic Metabolism in Stressful Exercise" published in January 2018 in *MOJ Sports Medicine*

Starting the training process by building a foundation prepares the body to tolerate more workload later in the season by means of:

- **Increased muscle efficiency.** Aerobic base training promotes the growth of mitochondria in muscle fibers, making them more efficient at using oxygen to produce energy. As a result of such training, the speed an athlete can maintain with easy effort will start to increase. In addition to that, mitochondria also process fatigue accumulated during high intensity training (by means of utilizing hydrogen ions), which is why higher mitochondrial density allows an athlete to process a greater training load and, as a result, see more improvement.

- **Increased efficiency of the cardiovascular system.** One of the positive side effects of aerobic training is an increase in the volume of the left ventricle of the heart. Together with increased blood plasma volume, it allows the heart to pump more blood to the working muscles and deliver more oxygen, while needing less beats (and energy) for it. This helps to provide the body with needed nutrients at low intensity and increases the maximum amount of oxygen the body can utilize at maximum effort (VO_2max). It's also why elite athletes have resting heart rate in the low or sub-40s.

- **Increased oxidation of fat.** Aerobic training improves the body's ability to burn fat for energy, which helps to preserve glycogen stores and operate more efficiently. On top of that, with proper nutrition it also results in a more athletic body composition (fat loss).

- **Reduced stress.** Low intensity training helps to activate the parasympathetic nervous system and allows the body to rest and recover more effectively. On top of that, high aerobic fitness correlates with reduced chronic inflammation, which further reduces the overall load on the body.

- **Reduced risk of injury.** Easy and prolonged exercise builds strength and resilience in structures that support our movement—stabilizing muscles, ligaments, and tendons—which are crucial in keeping the body aligned and injury-free. Individually, these structures are weaker than primary muscle groups and when fatigued, they do not operate effectively. So, when the training load is increased gradually, there's enough time for them to recover and grow stronger.

On the contrary, low aerobic fitness can have a detrimental effect on long-term health. In particular, Left Ventricular Hypertrophy (LVH) is a condition when the walls of the heart's main pumping chamber (left ventricle) thicken. LVH causes the size of the heart to increase but compared to the increase in volume (a result of extended low intensity training), it doesn't increase the heart's efficiency at supplying oxygen—only the ability to beat faster and pump the blood quicker. It simply forces the heart to beat faster, which causes more stress and prevents the person from relaxing fully.

Athletes who are starting their journey should be very careful with adding intensity into their training plan. A common mistake made by people who were not active throughout their life and don't have a large aerobic background is to jump into an intense training schedule and follow protocols that call for maximum output. That level of intensity can pose a risk for long-term health, as it promotes the thickening of the left ventricle's walls, much like heavy weights promote muscle building (hence the name hypertrophy).

Instead, focusing on foundation and aerobic fitness is a much more sustainable approach. In fact, people who engage in aerobic endurance sports (i.e., cross-country skiing, long-distance running, competitive cycling) have on average 4.3 to 8.0 years higher life expectancy than those who don't.[1] In other words, the more aerobically fit a person is, the longer he or she is expected to live. And the more adventure he or she can have throughout life.

FUNCTIONAL STRENGTH

Strength is the cornerstone of a well-balanced athlete, regardless of whether you are in a speed, power, or endurance-dominant sport. Nobody ever tells an athlete to run slower or throw weaker—it's always higher, faster, *stronger*. Becoming stronger has an impact on all areas of performance ability—it allows athletes to execute more powerful and controlled movements, maintain the form despite increasing fatigue, achieve greater speed, endure more, and also become more resilient to injuries during extensive training.

In short, strength training is a structured process of performing exercises against resistance with the goal to increase the body's ability to generate force and benefit performance. Overcoming a certain resistance that over time increases (progressive overload) provides

---

1   In reference to research titled "Does Physical Activity Increase Life Expectancy?" published on July 1, 2012, in *Journal of Aging Research*.

an external stimulus greater than that which the body would otherwise experience. That triggers adaptations in the muscle tissue and central nervous system (CNS) which make the body stronger and more efficient at recruiting the relevant muscles—just like during aerobic training.

Not all athletes are fans of strength training, though. Some avoid it out of fear of putting on too much muscle mass and getting slower. Others are concerned they might get injured, and there are those who are simply too focused on their primary activity (i.e., running, cycling, kayaking) and don't have extra time. However, if done right, strength training can become the secret sauce that elevates the athlete's performance to the next level—much more than an extra 30-minute run (or two).

Bodybuilder type of strength training is just one variation and is not really relevant for the majority of athletes due to the amount of recovery it requires. Effective strength training does not always result in muscle building. Its purpose for most athletes is to improve athletic performance, not necessarily increase size. That is, to develop power, improve maximum speed, promote muscle economy, reduce risk of injury, and even build endurance. Which is why to provide maximum effect, strength training should be functional and balanced across the following elements:

- **Flexibility and mobility** to increase the Range of Motion (ROM) of the joints and improve the body's ability to apply force. This type of training requires the use of muscle release techniques and easy exercises that utilize full ROM (i.e., shoulder or hip circles).

- **Injury prevention** strengthens joints and stabilizes muscles, as well as build resilience across the body against injuries during intense or prolonged training. It includes core and stabilizing exercises done at slow speeds to activate muscles and increase time under tension.

- **Movement quality and neuromuscular coordination** to ensure the body functions as a whole and can produce coordinated, efficient, and powerful movements. It requires the use of compound movement exercises (pushups, pullups, deadlifts, etc.), as well as constant repetition of the same movement pattern at low intensity to build a mind-body connection and optimize the form.

- **Strength and power** to produce more powerful movements and improve the efficiency of a particular activity by means of using less of the muscle's capacity. Such type of training requires sub-maximal resistance (i.e., squats or deadlifts with training load exceeding 80% of maximum) or harder variations of the exercise (i.e., pistol squat progression).

- **Metabolic conditioning** to improve the ability to maintain power for longer and develop muscular endurance. It requires increasing speed of execution and adding sport-specific movements. This can be achieved with popular boot camp workouts and timed circuit training.

Effective strength training focuses on mobility first to make sure the body is able to use the entire range of motion and operate at full potential. To that, athletes add components one by one, movement quality, injury prevention, maximum strength and metabolic conditioning. In doing so athletes should focus on their entire body—not just in one particular area. All muscles in the body are interlinked, so we never activate only one specific group. Even runners actively use their arms to balance and control the cadence and kayakers use their legs to turn their torso and produce a more powerful stroke.

CASE STUDY: BUILDING STRENGTH TO IMPROVE TRIATHLON PERFORMANCE

Norseman has the reputation of being the hardest triathlon on the planet. A race that organizers claim every hard-core triathlete should experience at least once is like an Iron-distance triathlon on steroids. Besides covering 140.6 miles (226.3K), athletes have to swim in the 57°F (14°C) water and climb over 16,400ft (5,000m) of vertical elevation during the bike and run leg. And for Hans, who reached out to me for coaching, racing in these kinds of events was, sort of, a hobby.

46 years old and a father of three kids, Hans was doing endurance sports throughout his entire life with the last 15 being focused on triathlon and trail running. Life outside training was pretty active as well with lots of skiing and hiking with the family. So, overall, a great example of a resilient athlete, yet he felt his body was getting older and was looking for a change in the approach.

Hans' training was already very consistent. Six days per week and roughly 10 hours of total volume gave him a very solid aerobic capacity. However, despite living in the mountainous region of Norway, cycling was not his strong suit and the second half of the run always gave him trouble due to the elevation gain throughout the race. Which is why the key change we made was his strength training approach. In particular, during winter he worked on maximum strength to improve the force he was producing and in spring he transitioned it into bike power and run fitness. That included:

- **Winter:** Two strength sessions per week focusing on heavy lifting with long rest and two core sessions per week to improve the body's ability to maintain the form
- **Spring:** Two low-cadence strength session on the bike to improve bike power and one plyometrics session to build resilience for the descents during the run section of the race

Early in the spring, Hans shared that he felt much more comfortable on the hills in the area he lived. Also, going for bike rides became more enjoyable, as it felt much easier. In fact, he timed himself on one of the climbs and found his personal best went down from 3 minutes and 41 second to 3 minutes and 9 seconds—a 15% improvement over a short distance while training for a 9-hour race. On top of that, he finished the Swedeman Tri (alternative to Norseman) that year in 8 hours and 56 minutes, which is 50 minutes faster than his best time 10 years earlier. And all of it from the change in the approach, not the volume.

Strength training has the potential to not only enhance sport-specific performance, but also raise the quality of life by means of improving the ability of individuals to do everyday activities, navigate chronic diseases, and even maintain good body composition. It is particularly relevant for 40+ athletes for whom strength training can reduce the magnitude of physical function decline associated with ageing. One of the effects is muscle mass loss of approximately 3–8%[1] per decade after the age of 30 (even higher after the age of 60), which reduces the functionality of a person and poses high risk of falling—a significant cause of age-related trauma. Another important variable is the reduced potential of the muscles and

---

1   In reference to the research titled "Muscle tissue changes with aging" published on January 12, 2010, in *Current Opinion in Clinical Nutrition and Metabolic Care*

high injury risk due to loss of mobility. The flexibility of the shoulder and hip joints decrease by ~6 degrees per decade after the age of 55.[1]

According to various research, a lot of the deterioration of the physical function associated with ageing can be attributed to a more sedentary lifestyle—not necessarily the process of ageing itself. Which is why staying fit and healthy and leading an active lifestyle is reliant on the maintenance of an exercise program. Consistent strength training can slow down physiological decline by means of increasing muscle mass and bone density, as well as enabling better balance and functionality for older adults.

SKILLS AND CONDITIONING

Athletes are defined not only by the "size of their engine," but also by how agile and skilled they are, how efficient their movements are and overall how resilient they are. While aerobic capacity and strength training will make an athlete more well-rounded, it is sport or adventure-specific skills and conditioning that will help him or her to produce the best performance. We can't "muscle" our way through lack of those skills. No matter how strong or fast we are, we won't be able to surf well if we can't swim or at least paddle properly. Or reach the summit of a technical mountain safely without advanced climbing skills.

While from the sidelines it might seem that hard workouts shape an athlete and get him or her fitter to tolerate more training load, it's actually the other way around. **The high level of base fitness that athletes accumulate over the years of practice is what helps them tolerate and improve more.** And that consists of the little things they do every day. The basics, like warmups, technique drills, skill practice, tactics (both in team sports and single events), basic and advanced conditioning exercises and even balance and coordination. Particularly when tired, stressed or not in the mood to do it. How many amateur athletes have that discipline?

Eventually, these small daily actions stack up one on top of another and create a snowball effect. Repeating movements hundreds of times over weeks, months and years helps athletes to improve technical mechanics and build strength in stabilizing muscles, which helps to create efficiency.

---

1   In reference to the study titled "Flexibility of Older Adults Aged 55–86 Years and the Influence of Physical Activity", published on June 19, 2013, in *Journal of Aging Research*

Practicing the skill in different conditions or under pressure (i.e., foreign environment or with elevated heart rate) is like adding resistance. It forces the body to grow and adapt more.

Simulating a certain experience in training helps condition the body to perform and builds the required skills for a particular activity. It also adds a touch of adventure to the process. Just like an athlete would adapt the training process for the demands of a marathon or triathlon (i.e., simulating effort, terrain, or impact of the long distance), he or she needs to adapt his training for the active lifestyle. Be it surfing different waves, being ready to trek for 12 hours a day or navigating varying terrains on a trail run, practice is necessary to be able to use our strength and aerobic capacity to the full extent.

However, as much as it's important to condition the body in the primary sport, it is equally important to challenge it to perform activities that it is less comfortable with. It's called cross training which is performing any physical activity that differs from an athlete's main one. Engaging in diverse activities activates and develops muscle groups that are otherwise less involved, which makes an athlete more balanced and resilient. It's also a great opportunity to relax both physically and mentally and use fitness for fun and pleasure.

Here are some ideas to include cross-training into the schedule:

- **Active recovery.** For an outsider, the phrase "recovery workout" might sound counter-intuitive, if not like total nonsense. But for athletes who cracked the code of high performance, it makes all the sense in the world. Cross-training can be a form of recovery, as long as athletes keep their effort fairly low. 30 to 60 minutes of very light (Zone 1 activity) helps to promote the blood flow across the body and relieve muscle tightness, which speeds up recovery.

- **Supportive workouts.** Cross-training can be used to maintain and even improve aerobic fitness. Cycling, for example, uses similar muscle groups that running does without putting excessive pressure on them, which makes it a great alternative for building an aerobic base. Swimming is another great way to cross-train, as it helps to strengthen supportive muscles, increase ankle flexibility, and improve body control, which promotes a more efficient running stride. Even something as simple as moving more (i.e., 10,000 steps per day) is a great way to make the body overall more resilient and able to tolerate more workload.

- **Balance and coordination activities.** A session of Pilates, Yoga, Tai Chi, or any other activity that improves body control is a great way to mobilize the muscles, as well as build the strength of stabilizing muscles. That helps to distribute stress evenly across the body, prevent injuries and improve form. It can also be a very powerful meditation tool once you get past the struggle to keep the posture.

- **Group activities.** Hiking, playing team or individual sports (volleyball, squash, etc.), going for social rides, all of these are a great way to socialize, do something new together and improve fitness. Take a group of friends and do something you haven't done before. Go explore a new route, climb a mountain or even try a new sport altogether. Immerse yourself in the moment and enjoy what your fitness enables you to do. After all, we tend to remember those moments the most, because that's when we feel we are living fully. Whenever I meet with my old friends, we still remember that 100k overnight kayak marathon that we did "for fun."

EXERCISE: HOW WELL-ROUNDED ARE YOU?

Is your training focused on squeezing out every bit of energy you have in order to maximize performance? Or are you training with the goal of staying active and in the best shape of your life for the years to come? Being a resilient athlete is not about adding as much training as possible. It's about organizing training and lifestyle so that the body is prepared to handle various demands and operate effectively in any situation. For that, a good indicator is how much fun you are having with your training.

For this exercise, you will need to evaluate your typical week and analyze how much variety is there in your schedule. It's best to take one of the previous weeks to avoid over- or underestimating the level and type of activity you engage in. Consider how you spend the week and use the quiz below to help you assess your lifestyle. Calculate your well-rounded-ness score on a weekly basis using the table below.

Note that a long training session totals just 1 point, even if it might be two or even three times longer than a short one. Same goes for high intensity sessions and any other activities, one point for each. That reflects the idea that being well-rounded and resilient is not about volume, but quality.

AEROBIC FITNESS	SCORE
Short and easy aerobic training (<1 hour)—*1 point for every session*	
Long and easy aerobic training (>1 hour)—*1 point for every session*	
Moderate intensity training (interval or sustained tempo)—*1 point for every session*	
High intensity training (interval or sustained tempo)—*1 point for every session*	
FUNCTIONAL STRENGTH	**SCORE**
Flexibility and mobility—*1 point for every activity (10+ minutes) that improves range of motion*	
Injury prevention—*1 point for every core or muscle stabilization activity (10+ minutes)*	
Movement quality—*1 point for every movement quality-related session (30+ minutes)*	
Strength and power—*1 point for every strength-focused session (30+ minutes)*	
Metabolic conditioning—*1 point for every intense strength conditioning session (30+ minutes)*	
SKILLS AND CONDITIONING	**SCORE**
Balance—*1 point for every balance-related activity (30+ minutes), like Yoga, Pilates, Tai Chi, etc.*	
Skill practice—*1 point for every focused drill or sport-specific skill practice (10+ minutes)*	
Group activities—*1 point for every game (30+ minutes) you engage in, like volleyball, squash, etc.*	
Cross training—*1 point for every extra activity (30+ minutes) you engage in, like hiking, SUP, etc.*	
Daily activity—*1 bonus point if you cover on average 10,000+ steps every day*	

0 to 7 points

That's barely scratching the surface. Your training is either too focused on one specific activity (i.e., only running or lifting weights) or you are not training enough. Consider splitting training into multiple sessions each with a different purpose, cross-training, adding different activities throughout the week and overall moving more.

8 to 14 points

It looks like you have good balance in your training process and you are on your way to being a well-rounded athlete. Most likely, you are very active throughout the week and across various activities. However, there's more potential for you to improve. To grow further, consider adding small elements to your daily routine, like core exercises, morning mobility practice, technique drills during easy sessions.

More than 15 points

Great job! Your training is balanced across various activities and your lifestyle outside of sports is quite active too. The quality you bring to the process via small elements helps to make the process ultra-effective. Keep up the good work.

Once you have the results, analyze what's missing and what you need to change in your training process to become more balanced. Define a specific goal and reorganize your week accordingly. The tools in the chapters ahead will help you do that: regulate intensity and recovery (Chapter 14), plan ahead (Chapter 15) and make the training process sustainable (Chapter 16).

BREAK THROUGH THE PLATEAU

Beast mode on. No pain no gain. *#workoutwednesday.*

There's a clear pattern one can spot when scrolling through the social media accounts of fitness enthusiasts. Their feeds are filled with impressive workouts that get hundreds of likes and reactions. It creates the impression that high intensity training (in the gym, on the track or anywhere else) is the answer to getting fit, strong, fast, gorgeous, and overall, a great athlete.

Unfortunately, with a go-go-go mentality many athletes fall into the pitfall of the so-called low return training. They go out for a run or a bike ride feeling they need to push themselves for the workout to count. Because, you know, a slow jog is not impressive. Fatigue or exhaustion makes them feel good about the job done and they do it again and again. Even though it makes an individual feel as if he or she is "working out," training like that every day is not too hard to effectively trigger neuromuscular adaptations and not easy enough to promote recovery or build endurance.

What ends up happening as a result of such low return training is that athletes consistently find themselves a little too tired. Always not to their 100%—both physically and mentally—and when it's time to go really hard they do not feel fully fresh and ready to do so. That has an effect on performance, outcome, productivity and even self-confidence. While there's a lot of talk about training more and harder (more intervals, longer duration, bootcamp this, Tabata that), there's very little about training smarter. Slowing down, focusing on quality, and being structured is not spectacular nor sexy…that is, until it produces the desired effect.

During coaching sessions, I frequently hear a message that sounds like this: "I'm struggling to get faster. I tried everything—more volume, different intervals, hill repeats, very long runs, strength training—but nothing seems to work. Can you help?" Unfortunately, it's a situation many amateur and self-coached athletes find themselves in. Not seeing expected results is frustrating. It drains self-confidence and prompts people to switch from program to program in a search for a winning strategy to overcome the training plateau, often with little success.

No, these athletes are not broken or destined to participate in the competitions only as spectators. And yes, there is still hope that they can change things for the better. Personally, I'm always excited for these messages, because it means a person is open to changing his or her existing habits and is driven by growth. There is usually a single tweak that a person needs to make for things to start falling into places: intensity.

Every adaptation in the body—endurance, speed, power and even muscle growth—is triggered by a specific intensity level and requires a certain amount to be effective. Call it a recipe: if you add too much or too little of a particular ingredient, the result will not be as expected. Dialing in the intensity is how elite athletes maintain progress while many self-coached athletes get stuck in a training plateau. It is the key factor that makes any training program fit and often what self-coached athletes misjudge…and as a result, causes them not to see their expected results.

The way to break through the plateau is to focus on quality and make sure the intensity of every training session is dialed in. You don't need to remember hundreds of different workouts. Nor do you need to test multiple training plans and jump from one fitness trend to the next until you find the one that fits. In this chapter, I will share the principles behind the training intensity so that you can start introducing them into your training process and improving its quality. All you need to do is become aware of what every training session is set to accomplish, select the right recipe from the cookbook and add it into your routine.

SUPERCOMPENSATION

Our bodies go through a certain degree of stress while exercising, which is known as training load. Regardless of whether that load is high (i.e., hard intervals, racing) or low (i.e., a session of Yoga or easy cycling), additional demand placed on the body decreases its physical capabilities. Once the exercise is over, the body starts to actively bring all systems back to normal. Repair micro tears in the muscle tissue. Restock energy and nutrient supplies. Calm down the nervous system. Utilize the hormones that were released in response to stress.

Recovery time is where it gets exciting. The body doesn't just bounce back to the same physical condition it was in before the training session. It is smart and grows a little stronger in response to the physical stimuli to ensure that when the same stress occurs next time, the body will be able to tolerate it better. **This adaptation to a more intense effort (or more training volume) is called the supercompensation effect.** When it occurs, an athlete is able to perform better and process more training load, which, ultimately, helps to become even stronger, faster and more enduring.

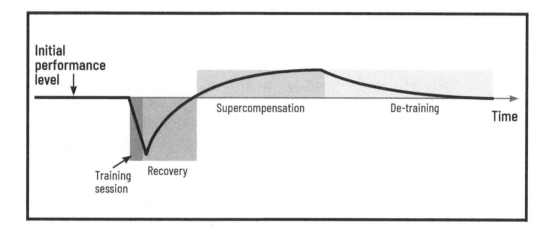

Illustration of the supercompensation effect following a training practice.

The magnitude of the supercompensation effect depends on the training load. The more the body goes through, the greater the effect. That holds true for both the immediate supercompensation (following a training practice) and a long-term one (following a training block). However, increased performance ability lasts from a few days to a week after which the body starts to de-train and lose fitness if not stimulated further. Which is why the timing of the training practice is very important. If the next key session (one that is focused on improving fitness) takes place when the body is not in the most optimal condition (recovering or de-training), performance will not improve as expected.

Let's take an example of when an athlete recovers for too long. Amanda is a typical hobby runner who trains two to three times per week for around 20–30 minutes. When she started running a few years ago, exercising three times per week helped her shed some post-pregnancy weight and improve endurance to the extent that she could cover 5K without stopping. However, since then the progress has slowed down and she didn't improve much. This is a common situation many newcomer athletes face: they don't train frequently enough. Sometimes they do a good session, but then life happens, and they skip anywhere from a few days to a few weeks. By the time they are back at it, the body is, most probably, down to its initial performance level.

Putting the body through the same training load allows it to adapt only to a certain level. To grow further, it has to be challenged more.

Fixed intensity, lack of intense workouts, or training sessions far apart from each other are not challenging the body enough to make a substantial leap. This doesn't provide enough stimulus for the body and instead lets it enter the de-training state and allows fitness to slide back to its initial level. In a longer perspective, such sporadic training does not result in a significant fitness gain.

Competitive athletes have the opposite problem. **They tend to overestimate how fit they can get in the near future and underestimate how long the recovery from a particular training session will take.** Many try to copy training programs from elite athletes or complete very hard sessions which their bodies do not recover as quickly from. For example, a 2-hour run or an intense VO$_2$max session can provide a lot of training benefits, but an athlete who has not yet developed aerobic fitness will stay sore and tired (if not injured or down with a cold) for the next few days, which will impact the rest of the training week. For this athlete, it's more effective to have many easier sessions than a few major ones. When a key training session takes place while the body is still recovering, fatigue will accumulate and the body's readiness to perform will diminish.

Plateaus or even declines in performance can also happen when an athlete has been pushing things too much for too long. There is a misconception that low intensity exercise is not effective and non-professional athletes should train harder to compensate for lack of time. However, it usually results in an unstructured approach and too much time spent training at intensity that is comfortably uncomfortable—hard enough to feel like you are exercising, but not hard enough to make a meaningful shift in fitness. In many cases, athletes spend months and years in this plateau, unaware they are slowly burning out. They don't allow themselves to recover fully and because of that, miss out on most of the benefits from their training.

Incomplete recovery and the state of constant exhaustion some athletes experience paired with overall stress, can result in a so-called adrenal depletion: a condition where the adrenal glands are no longer able to maintain proper hormone levels and athletic performance is severely compromised. **In simple words, it means overtraining.** It happens when the body has been producing excessive amounts of cortisol (in response to stress) for an extended period of time, forcing the adrenal glands to work without getting a chance to rest and "recharge." When they get taxed too much for too long, their ability to maintain even normal levels of cortisol becomes impaired. The result? Tremendous fatigue, sometimes for no apparent reason. Workout splits get slower. It gets harder to get out of bed. An athlete feels tired even after a rest day or having no energy despite sleeping for over 10 hours.

Some other symptoms include:

- Lack of appetite or cravings for salty and sweet foods
- Muscle soreness or "heaviness"
- Loss of enjoyment for sport
- Depression or general loss of motivation
- Moodiness and irritability
- Loss of sex drive

It's not hard training that makes athletes fitter, but the recovery from it—that critical period when the body grows stronger and adapts to a higher workload. If recovery is not sufficient, athletes risk accumulating more fatigue and compromising all the effort they are putting in. To prevent this debilitating situation, they should aim to completely recover on a constant basis to ensure the body super-compensates. Timing key training sessions and buildup weeks to when the body is at its strongest helps to tolerate more training load and in that way, break through the training plateau. It also adds small checkpoints along the way that can be used to measure fitness gains.

In practice, it's not necessary to super-compensate for each and every session. The training plan should resemble an upward spiral where an athlete puts the most stress on the body (key training session) when it's capacity to perform is at its highest and then reduces the workload (through rest days, recovery or supportive sessions) in the following days. This gives the body time to adapt to the training load and in the next cycle tolerate even more.

There are lots of factors influencing recovery and some of these we cannot control. Daily stress, past training and even weather—anything that impacts an athlete's performance also impacts recovery. Which is why the best approach is to listen to the body and use that to make decisions about training workload and rest (refer to Chapter 9 for strategies). More often than not, It's better to switch training days to allow the body to achieve optimal condition. Here are some cues to look for:

- **Heart rate.** Consistent aerobic training results in the increase of the heart's size and the development of a capillary network. This makes the blood transport across the body more efficiently and reduces the heart rate. A similar effect happens during supercompensation: as the body adapts to an increase in training load, both the resting heart rate and heart rate during the training session (at a specific pace) decreases.

- **Performance gains.** When the body adapts to the training load, there are obvious performance gains. Athletes may notice that the previous effort feels easier, they are able to reach higher speeds or even lift more. This effect is the same across all sports: running, cycling, weightlifting, you name it.

- **Energy and mood.** When athletes are fully recovered, they feel more energetic and in general are in a much better mood. And not only that, their productivity increases, they complain less and, generally, tend to enjoy life more.

Making changes to the training process on the go based on the feedback the body provides is where training zones become handy. They help to vary the training, tailor it for specific needs and make sure the body is in optimal condition to improve.

BUILDING AEROBIC FITNESS WITH ZONE TRAINING

Training without considering the exact intensity that each session requires is like navigating a ship without a compass. You may get where you want to, but it won't be smooth sailing.

Sounds reckless, but that is a mistake many athletes make. They follow a plan that doesn't specify how hard to train and end up getting varying results from trial and error. **Correct intensity is what brings quality to the process and makes each session purposeful—be it improving power, endurance, speed or even recovering.** Pacing yourself to exercise at the right effort does require patience and a great deal of self-regulation, which is why developing physical resilience is highly dependent on the balance across other resilience domains.

Each effort level (measured as a share of maximum output) triggers different physiological processes in our body, which has an impact on the kind of adaptation effect that will take place as a result. Training zones help to categorize those adaptations, so that athletes can customize their training and tailor it for specific needs. Moreover, training in zones prevents situations where results start to stagnate because an athlete runs too fast or too slow. Training zones focus on the effort, not on a certain pace. So, when the athlete's physical condition changes, his or her pace for a certain zone will also change and will continue to provide further stimulus to adapt more; for example, when an athlete becomes fitter his running pace for Zone 2 also increases.

Focusing each training session around a specific intensity zone helps to target specific adaptations that help an athlete improve a certain attribute: aerobic base, power, speed, etc. That is sometimes referred to as "training in zones."

Let's look at an example to visualize the concept of training zones better. Consider Ben, a 30-year-old man who has been running actively for the past 3 years and wants to use a more scientific approach to improve his fitness. He has signed up to do a supervised VO_2max test in a laboratory to determine his current level of fitness and areas he should improve in. The test used progressive intensity protocol (increasing speed by +0.3 km/h every minute) to determine the body's maximum capabilities. It started at very low intensity (leisurely walking pace) and for the first several minutes, Ben didn't feel as if he was exercising at all.

However, after switching to a jog he felt his breathing intensified. As the speed increased further, inhaling got deeper and soon breathing exclusively through the nose became impossible. Several more minutes later, the speed got so fast that Ben started to gasp for air and felt his muscles tensing up. He pushed himself for a few more minutes until his legs couldn't keep up and forced him to stop.

During the test Ben was asked to wear a mask that measured the volume of carbon dioxide he exhaled at every point of time. On top of that, assistants took blood samples from his finger at the beginning of every minute to determine the level of lactate the muscles accumulated. The purpose of all of that was to determine two specific points of time when Ben's physiology changed: aerobic and anaerobic thresholds.

- **Aerobic threshold** was the first point of time when Ben's breathing intensified. It is the intensity level after which the body turns on the anaerobic system and starts to (very slowly) accumulate lactate; i.e., the muscles begin to fatigue. It is barely noticeable, as the rate of that accumulation is not yet high. If the speed remained constant, Ben could have continued jogging like that for hours.

- **Anaerobic threshold** occurred when Ben started to gasp for air and felt his muscles getting heavy. Until that time even though he was already running fast, the body was able to process some of the lactate that had built up. Had the speed remained the same, Ben could have continued for longer, but as it increased further, lactate started to accumulate quicker, and the body was not able to process it anymore. His muscles tensed up and he was forced to stop within a few minutes.

Aerobic and anaerobic thresholds correlate to a certain level of lactate in our blood that is produced in response to particularly hard (or long) exercise. Physiologically, during strenuous muscle activity the body produces large amounts of waste products that need to be removed to continue. Most notably, hydrogen ions ($H+$) that cause muscle "heaviness" and carbon dioxide (CO_2) that intensifies the breathing.

Accumulation of such waste reduces our body's pH level (creates an acidic state), causes the lactate level to grow exponentially and limits our performance ability. The body will, essentially, start to "shut down" to prevent damaging itself because it cannot sustain such toxicity. If you have ever pushed yourself to the point of exhaustion (or ran 400 meters all-out), you'll know how this works in practice—breathing very hard, muscles feel like stones and can hardly move, head spinning.

Both thresholds are important but have their own specifics. In particular, the higher the aerobic threshold the faster an athlete can run, bike, kayak or perform any other cyclical activity without accumulating much fatigue. That is the athlete's general endurance. On top of that, a high aerobic threshold means muscles contain a lot of mitochondria, which helps the body to process fatigue and, as a result, impacts how much high intensity an athlete can sustain at a time. The common problem that athletes face is that they don't build a solid aerobic base (improve aerobic threshold much) and, therefore, have less capacity to perform high intensity training.

On the other hand, training around the anaerobic threshold will make muscles more resistant to lactate build up and reduce the rate at which it accumulates during a very intense activity. This helps to maintain very high speed for longer, which is critical for short races and performances (lasting up to 5 minutes).

For aerobic training to be effective, every effort should focus on either of the two effects: pushing the aerobic threshold further (through volume and mostly lower intensity) or changing the angle of the anaerobic threshold (by using intervals at or around the threshold). Training zones are organized around these thresholds to help target the required effect and provide just enough stimulus to ensure supercompensation. However, each zone has a certain recipe (duration and rest) in order to be effective, so when planning a session, it is important to consider that. Doing so produces exceedingly effective results, even at low training volumes. Not as simple as picking a workout from the magazine and smashing yourself, is it?

ZONE	ADAPTATIONS	PURPOSE	MIN. DURATION FOR ADAPTATION
Zone 1	Promotes blood flow. Prolonged efforts over time increase levels of blood plasma and blood stroke volume, resulting in better cardiac efficiency.	Active recovery, warm-up, cool down, aerobic base	Multiple hours (for aerobic benefit) or <40min for active rest and recovery
Zone 2	Builds general endurance and resilience across the body to be able to exercise for long duration. Fitness gains are long-lasting. **Race effort for events lasting 6+ hours**	Aerobic base (easy pace)	30+ minutes
Zone 3	Develops aerobic capacity and muscle economy to be able to maintain moderate efforts for longer. **Race effort for events lasting 3–6 hours**	Aerobic capacity (tempo/steady pace)	Long intervals (10+ minutes)
Zone 4	Develops aerobic power and capacity, as well as cruising speed at lactate threshold effort. Used to develop power in base period, as well as for race-specific training. **Race effort for events lasting 45 minutes—3 hours**	Aerobic capacity and power (lactate threshold)	Medium-length intervals (1–10 minutes)
Zone 5a	Improves maximum oxygen capacity and utilization, as well as develops muscular endurance. **Race effort for events lasting 10—45 minutes**	VO_2max	Short intervals (~1min)
Zone 5b	Builds anaerobic capacity and power, as well as improves lactate tolerance—ability of the body to utilize lactate for energy. **Race effort for events lasting up to 10 minutes**	Anaerobic capacity	Short intervals (~20–40sec)
Zone 5c	Develops ability of the body to recruit muscle fibers more effectively, thereby improving maximum speed. **Sprint race effort**	Neuro-muscular power	Short intervals (>10sec)

Summary of training zones and their effect on the body.

Zone 1: Recovery/Warm-up

Zone 1 is the exercise intensity up to the level of the aerobic threshold. Notice how the lactate in the graph decreases in the first few minutes of the test. That is because the intensity of the exercise is so low that the small amount of already accumulated lactate from daily activities is being actively utilized. Active rest helps muscles to bounce back quicker. Studies found that the lactate utilization post intense exercise is 48% faster[1] following recovery efforts than after passive rest. Moving the body also promotes blood flow and activates the lymphatic system, which makes Zone 1 perfect for recovery (after harder training sessions or in between intervals).

Moreover, at aerobic threshold the volume of blood that the heart pumps out is at its maximum. Beyond that point, it's only the heart rate that increases—not the stroke volume. Which is why spending an extended amount of time in Zone 1 "stretches" the left ventricle of the heart and increases the efficiency of the cardiovascular system. In fact, professional athletes (regardless of the race distance) usually start their season with a 3–4-week-long training camp where they focus primarily on Zones 1 and 2. Every day they would put in 5–6 hours of easy work to train the heart, focus on the form, as well as work on the base muscle strength.

Below are some of the examples of how Zone 1 can be used in the training process:

- Warmup, cool down and recovery between repeats during interval session
- Short recovery sessions of up to 40 mins
- Long base-building sessions of 2+ hours

---

1   In reference to the study titled "Effect of Active Versus Passive Recovery on Performance During Intrameet Swimming Competition" published on August 19, 2013, in *Sports Health*.

Zone 2: Aerobic Base

Zone 2 is the exercise intensity just above the aerobic threshold. It's still considered low intensity; exercising in this zone feels so easy that those who are new to such training may feel as though they are not training hard enough. Athletes tend to be surprised at how slowly they need to go to stay within Zone 2 and often have a hard time overcoming the idea that sometimes they have to slow down to a walk to do that. However, the benefits of low intensity training (base strength, endurance, and resilience across the body) come from volume and consistency, not from exhaustion.

The goal in Zone 2 training is to exercise at a pace that allows an athlete to sustain easy effort for a prolonged time period (30+ minutes). Pushing the body to go for a little longer helps the body to become more efficient over time. Physiologically what happens is oxidative muscle fibers (high concentration of mitochondria—slow-twitch) start to fatigue and glycolytic (low concentration of mitochondria—fast-twitch) begin to take over the load. Activation of these fibers promotes the growth of mitochondria in them, which makes them more efficient. As a result, the athlete becomes faster while still exercising at an easy pace. On top of that, extended easy training teaches the body to utilize fat better and improves oxygen transport.

For non-professional athletes, one of the most efficient ways to significantly improve fitness is to increase the overall volume and Zone 2 training provides good framework for that. It ensures that most of the volume is done at low intensity and is not too stressful for the body to handle. This, in turn, develops a solid aerobic base and prevents burnout that could be caused by more intense sessions. Moreover, since mitochondria grow within 24 hours, Zone 2 sessions don't require a lot of recovery time (unless they are extra-long) and athletes can even include multiple of these in a day.

Below are some of the examples of how Zone 2 can be used in the training process:

- Long base-building sessions of 60+ minutes
- Aerobic "maintenance" sessions of 30 to 60 minutes

STRATEGY: NASAL BREATHING

Athletes use various gadgets to measure many aspects of their training and lifestyle: exercise intensity, quality of sleep, running efficiency and so on. However, breathing is one piece of data that is not captured by any of the devices yet provides valuable information.

The way we breathe during exercise is a good indicator of how intense it is. In particular, Zones 2 and 3 can be very hard to distinguish, even when a person is using a heart rate monitor to control the intensity. Because of the similarities between the two effort levels athletes might find themselves exercising just a little too hard for optimal adaptation. This is where paying attention to the breathing pattern can help you to stay on track:

- **Zone 2:** Athletes should be able to inhale and exhale exclusively through the nose. The occasional exhale through the mouth is not a problem.
- **Zone 3:** Breathing becomes deeper and athletes typically start exhaling through the mouth to help remove carbon dioxide quicker.
- **Zone 4:** Breathing intensifies even further and athletes start using mouth breathing more actively (for both inhaling and exhaling).

This difference in breathing patterns happens because the nose creates resistance to air flow (to warm up the air and stop bacteria from penetrating the body). It is harder to take in the air through the nose quickly, so when the intensity increases and the body requires more oxygen, breathing through the mouth becomes a natural reflex. However, even though the speed of breathing is slower when inhaling and exhaling exclusively through the nose, it allows more oxygen to be absorbed into the bloodstream.[1] On top of that, overcoming resistance that the nose creates, strengthens respiratory muscles and allows the body to capture oxygen more effectively (see the part about oxygenation in Chapter 10).

A great start is to practice nasal breathing during longer sessions to make sure you are exercising at low intensity and not over-exerting yourself. This will help to improve aerobic base, as well as train respiratory muscles to become more effective.

_____

1   In reference to the research titled "Effect of Nasal Versus Oral Breathing on Vo2max and Physiological Economy in Recreational Runners Following an Extended Period Spent Using Nasally Restricted Breathing." published on April 30, 2018, in the International Journal of Kinesiology and Sports Science.

Zone 3: Aerobic Capacity

Our body becomes more efficient (enduring) when we build mitochondria in glycolytic (fast-twitch) muscle fibers. However, as the aerobic base increases, the effect of Zone 2 training takes place later. Muscles fatigue slower, so in order to continue improving athletes need to train longer. In fact, for a triathlete who is preparing for an Ironman triathlon the training effect of a 4-hour-long bike ride will, most probably, take place in the last hour—the first three are required to set the body up for it to occur.

As you can imagine, when an athlete can comfortably perform for around 1.5 hours at Zone 2 intensity, it gets impractical to add more volume—both due to time commitment and potential impact on the joints as a result of continuous impact (i.e., during running). Luckily, long, and easy training is not the only way to improve endurance. Otherwise, we would have to train for hours every day to simply maintain fitness. Moderate and even high intensity intervals performed not until exhaustion also stimulate growth of mitochondria, which makes Zone 3 a very powerful tool for developing endurance.

Combining long easy training with some moderate efforts can simulate the effect of a longer session. In response, the body builds even more mitochondria, which leads to improved muscle economy and makes those moderate race efforts (half marathons, marathons, and even half-Ironman distance triathlons) feel easier and manageable.

Aerobic capacity improves when we challenge our aerobic energy system. Not to our physiological limit (i.e., all-out sprint), but only to the point where the anaerobic energy system takes over and lactate starts to accumulate quicker.

Zone 3 is the intensity level between aerobic and anaerobic thresholds and feels uncomfortable enough for an athlete to feel like he or she is exercising. At this intensity the breathing deepens and an athlete is barely able to complete a sentence before catching a breath, compared to conversational Zone 1 and 2 efforts. As a result, this intensity trains the body to consume and utilize oxygen better, thereby improving aerobic capacity. Such moderate efforts also engage more muscle fibers than Zone 2 training does, while producing less lactate than Zone 4. However, some athletes do make the mistake of spending the majority of their training time in this zone and, as a result, do not have the energy left to add higher intensity training that will improve top speed. This is the reason why Zone 3 got the reputation of being The No Man's Land—athletes push themselves, but do not necessarily get faster. The key to effective Zone 3 training is to use an interval method with short rest in between, instead of maintaining the effort throughout the entire session.

Below are some of the examples of how Zone 3 can be used in the training process:

- 3×15 minutes in low-Zone 3 during a long (60+ minutes) easy Zone 1–2 session
- 4×8 minutes in high-Zone 3 with 3-minute breaks in Zone 2
- Long tempo efforts (40 to 75 minutes) as a standalone session (for advanced athletes only)

Zone 4: Aerobic Capacity and Power

From a physiological standpoint, anaerobic threshold is the maximum intensity that the body can maintain while still utilizing oxygen. Training around this threshold improves the body's ability to utilize lactate for energy more effectively and, as a result, improves resistance to fatigue during very intense efforts. This state is known as muscular endurance. Training in this zone is particularly important for middle distance runners, kayakers, and swimmers, those whose race distance generally takes less than 4–5 minutes to complete. However, endurance athletes will also benefit from this kind of training, as it puts a high load on the aerobic energy system (thereby increasing aerobic capacity), builds power in muscles and makes longer distance running speed feel easier.

Training around or above the anaerobic threshold is very taxing on the body and of all five training zones, Zone 4 is the most sensitive to fatigue. Threshold sessions are very uncomfortable and cause, among other things, shortness of breath and acute muscle stiffness. Such training is only effective when the body is fully recovered and since many athletes are in a state of chronic fatigue, they dread or stay away from these very hard sessions. And as a result, do not train to their full potential.

Efforts done at the anaerobic threshold provide a lot of fitness benefits, but the way they are usually done (20–40-minute tempo efforts) requires a lot of recovery afterwards. A more effective way to train is to cut the total effort into smaller chunks and add short breaks in between. For the threshold to improve, the most important factor is the total time spent around threshold effort, so by allowing the body to recover a little, it is possible to increase the number of intervals and with that the total time at threshold. Instead of a 20-minute Zone 4 tempo a much more effective session would be to do 5×5-minute (25 minutes in total) threshold intervals and include 2-minute Zone 1 aerobic efforts in between.

While it is tempting to go all out during threshold sessions, the trick is to avoid complete exhaustion and instead stay within the prescribed 80%—90% effort range, always leaving a little more left in the tank.

The goal of Zone 4 training is not to run every interval at maximum speed, but rather to maintain the same hard effort throughout all repetitions. Think of it as splitting a longer distance into smaller chunks and adding short recoveries in between (like splitting 5K distance into 5x1K efforts). That way, you will be able to run every interval at a speed just slightly over one you would maintain for the full distance and gradually train the body to hold it for longer.

As this kind of training builds a lot of fatigue, start adding Zone 4 training only after building a solid aerobic base (at least 20 hours of aerobic activity). Mitochondria developed as a result of low intensity training will speed up recovery and allow the body to tolerate more training load.

Below are some of the examples of how Zone 4 can be used in the training process:

- Three sets of 3×2 minutes in Zone 4 with 1 minute recovery in Zone 1 (3 minutes recovery in Zone 1 between sets)
- 6×4 minutes in Zone 4 with 3 minutes recovery in Zone 1
- 12×1 minute in high-Zone 4 with 1 minute recovery in Zone 1

Zone 5: VO$_2$max, Anaerobic Capacity and Speed Training

Zone 5 is the "all-out" effort, the absolute maximum that your muscles can deliver. At this intensity, massive amounts of lactate are produced and it is impossible for the body to process it in time. Regardless of how good an athlete is, top speed can only be maintained for a brief period of time before muscles get very tight and heavy, forcing an athlete to slow down. At this effort, he or she is also breathless—there is no way to speak even a full word.

A typical Zone 5 effort ranges anywhere from 5 to 40 seconds and utilizes the combination of ATP/CP (stored energy) and lactic energy systems to produce training effects. The shorter the interval, the more intense the effort and the more ATP/CP energy system is used. Maximum intensity activates all (or nearly all) muscle fibers and rather than training the effectiveness of the energy system, it helps to build neural connections to muscle fibers and makes athletes better at activating them. That, in turn, translates to higher maximum speed and better muscle efficiency, which is the reason why athletes incorporate explosive exercises and short pickups to maximum speed (strides) in their sessions. For the same reason, Zone 5 training is great for practicing take-off speed (for race starts) and improving reaction time.

Moreover, since maximum intensity utilizes all muscle fibers, there is also an endurance benefit to it. If duration of the exercise is very short and includes a long rest interval, such training promotes growth of mitochondria in glycolytic (fast-twitch) muscle fibers and contributes to improving athlete's endurance.

Maximum effort training should be done using effort as a measure of intensity, not heart rate. Often, the heart rate doesn't even increase above 90% throughout most of the training session. However, it is a great way to check if the body has recovered from the intervals. As soon as the heart rate can't drop to Zones 1–2 after three minutes of rest, it's time to end the workout.

Below are some of the examples of how Zone 5 can be used in the training process:

- 5 sets of 3×20 seconds in Zone 5 with 20 second recovery in Zone 1 (5min recovery in Zone 1 between sets)
- 10×40 seconds in Zone 5 with 3-minute recovery in Zone 1
- 4 sets of 10-second bursts at close to maximum effort followed by 50 seconds in Zone 1 (5min recovery in Zone 1 between sets)

ZONE	EFFORT	BREATH/TALK TEST	RPE	%HRR
Zone 1	**Light**—hardly any exertion (feels 'effortless'). Could continue all day	Normal talking and breathing	1	<60%
Zone 2	**Easy**—gentle effort, but non-taxing. Could easily continue for hours	Becoming aware of the breath, but no issue holding a full conversation	2	60–70%
Zone 2	**Comfortable**—starting to feel the effort, but no problem to maintain it for an hour (or more)	Breathing becomes slightly deeper, but still possible entirely through the nose. Can say a few sentences	3	60–70%
Zone 3	**Moderate**—requires extra effort, but feels 'manageable'	Breathing entirely through the nose becomes difficult. Having difficulty completing long sentences	4	70–80%
Zone 3	**Comfortably uncomfortable**—effort starts to become challenging. *3:30+ marathon effort*	Breathing deepens and becomes more rhythmic. Conversing is only possible in short sentences	5	70–80%
Zone 4	**Vigorous**—feeling how the body is doing intense work. *Sub-3–hour marathon effort*	Breathing is deep and uncomfortable. Possible to speak 4–6 words at once	6	80–90%
Zone 4	**Hard**—becomes very uncomfortable to continue. *Half-marathon race effort*	Gasping for air after a few words. Not possible to maintain a conversation	7	80–90%
Zone 5	**Very hard**—feels difficult to maintain and requires focus to continue. *10K race effort*	Breathing is rapid, possible to speak a word or two at once.	8	>90%
Zone 5	**'Impossible'**—feels too fast and requires digging deep. *1K to 5K race effort*	Nearly breathless. Possible to make grunting sounds or spit out one-syllable words	9	n/a*
Zone 5	**Maximum effort**—says it all. Not possible to maintain for longer than 20–30 seconds	Breathless, gasping for air	10	n/a*

*Efforts that improve anaerobic capacity and power are typically very short and are done at close to full speed. It doesn't make sense to pace these efforts using heart rate, because it doesn't climb as fast.

*Training zone breakdown across two measurement methods: Rate of Perceived Exertion scale (RPE column) and percentage of Heart Rate Reserve (%HRR column).

HOW TO DETERMINE TRAINING ZONES

There are two main methods to determine training zones: Rate of Perceived Exertion (RPE) and the Heart Rate method. Both have their pros and cons, so it is best to cross-check one against the other to make sure you are exercising at the correct intensity.

Rate of Perceived Exertion is an old-school method. It is easy and it works well for people who are more in tune with their bodies. The RPE scale rates the intensity of the exercise from 1 to 10 based on how difficult it feels. Every effort level on the scale has specific cues and corresponds to a certain training zone, which makes it relatively easy to control the intensity of the exercise. Many top-level athletes use this method (consciously or not) primarily because they have vast experience and knowledge about how their bodies respond to the workload. Nonetheless, it is a great first step for any athlete to start learning how different training zones feel and affect the body.

The Rate of Perceived Exertion method has its limitations, mainly because every person has a different pain threshold or may experience the effort differently. For some, a certain intensity can feel like a 7, whereas for another it is more like a 5. In addition to that, reviewing the session after a longer period of time is very difficult because there is very limited reference of how the body responded throughout the exercise (i.e., how each interval felt or how tired the body got towards the end of the session).

A more precise and convenient way to use zones is to use the heart rate as a guide. The higher the training intensity the faster the heart needs to beat to move the blood to the working muscles. Moreover, as already discussed in Chapter 9, the heart rate is a very versatile parameter and reflects all stress factors that affect the body on a particular day: sleep quality, weather, impact of previous training, etc. We can do an all-out sprint set or not get enough sleep one night and see our heart rate going wild the next morning. This is why the use of heart rate training zones helps an athlete to ensure he or she is exercising at the right intensity given the current condition.

A training zone refers to a defined range (i.e., 60–70%), but it's not as straightforward as a percentage of maximum heart rate. Individual heart rate differs from person to person, which is why a so-called Target Heart Rate Zone formula developed by Finnish exercise physiologist, Martti Karvonen, is a more precise way of estimating zones. It is created based on thousands of people's laboratory test results and takes into account both maximum and resting heart rates that reflect an athlete's current fitness condition.

Target Heart Rate = [Max HR—Rest HR] * XX% + Rest HR

Max HR is the maximum number of beats the heart can perform under maximum stress and is an estimate of the maximum level of intensity an athlete can sustain. The easiest way to determine maximum heart rate would be to estimate it using a formula. While it may not be 100% precise, it's still a good start for those who are just starting out:

- [220—age] Most common and widely used maximum heart rate formula
- [207—0.7 × age] More precise formula, adjusted for people over the age of 40
- [211—0.64 × age] Slightly more precise formula, adjusted for generally active people

Unfortunately, none of the above-mentioned formulas are gender-adjusted. Generally, women tend to have a 5–10 beat higher heart rate than men, so that's something to account for.

Estimating your maximum heart rate can be biased because formulas generalize people and tend to be imprecise for very fit athletes and people of older age who are very active. And that is because efficiency of our heart muscle decreases with age (as it happens with any muscle in our body), which, in turn, results in decrease of maximum and sub maximum heart rates. However, athletes who maintain consistent training regime and engage in both low- and high-intensity exercise keep their heart muscle "conditioned," thereby slowing down the rate of decline.

If you have seen your heart rate go higher than what the formula suggests (like in a race or a time trial), do use that. In fact, experienced athletes (with aerobic background and a clearance from a physician) would be better off measuring their real maximum heart rate in a lab or by performing one of the field tests:

- 20-minute time trial
- 4×2min all-out intervals with 1 minute recovery
- Partner-assisted stress test (increasing the heart rate by 5 bpm every 15 seconds)

Rest HR is the heart rate at complete rest and is an estimate of current fitness. It can be observed first thing in the morning (before rolling out of bed) or after 2–3 minutes of laying rest. Heart rate can jump a couple of bpm from day to day depending on how well-rested you are, so use the average for the week in calculation.

Calculating target heart rate zones is about putting correct (and honest) numbers in the right places. Let's use Ben's example to visualize it. He measured his resting heart rate to be 50 bpm and estimated his maximum heart rate to be 192 bpm (using the 211—0.64 x Age formula). Putting in the numbers for Zone 2 resulted in:

A 60% effort equals [192—50] × 60% + 50 = 135 bpm

A 70% effort equals [192—50] × 70% + 50 = 149 bpm

So, if Ben wants to build a solid aerobic base (Target Heart Rate of 60–70%), he should make sure his heart rate stays between 135 and 149 beats per minute during his long base-building efforts.

BUILDING STRENGTH WITH RESISTANCE AND VELOCITY

Strength training shouldn't be focused on getting bigger muscles because it's what we can do with them that counts. It doesn't make much sense to have big muscles and see them covered in fat or get fatigued quickly. There's more to strength and conditioning than simply lifting weights. When the process is structured to produce supercompensation, not add more fatigue, it has a substantial effect on an athlete's performance and the quality of life. To maximize results from training efforts, every session has to target specific adaptations. Much like aerobic training should vary to prevent training plateau, there is a certain progression in strength training as well.

Strength training doesn't follow the zone methodology, because almost every activity involves overcoming resistance and is much shorter in duration than aerobic training. As a result, every effort is essentially a high intensity one. However, strength training also requires variety and structure to be effective and that quality is achieved through controlling the speed of execution (velocity), load (resistance) and the rest interval. By manipulating these factors, athletes can trigger different adaptations: build neural pathways, grow mitochondria in the muscle tissue, or build muscle.

TYPE OF TRAINING	OUTCOME	RECIPE
Anatomical Adaptation	Base strength	Load: bodyweight (add if necessary) Speed of execution: slow to moderate Repetitions: 15–20 (until discomfort) Rest: minimum (30–60sec)
Hypertrophy	Muscle size	Load: 60%—80% of 1RM Speed of execution: slow eccentric, fast concentric Repetitions: 6–12 per set, until failure Rest: 2–5min between sets
Maximum Strength	Maximum force	Load: 80%—90% of 1RM Speed of execution: explosive Repetitions: 1–3 per set Rest: 3–5min between sets
Power Development	Sport-specific strength	Load: up to 50% of 1RM Speed of execution: explosive Repetitions: 3–6 per set Rest: 2–3min
	Muscular endurance	Load: 30%—50% of 1RM Speed of execution: fast Time: 1–4 min Rest: 15sec (exercise), 2–4 min (circuit)

Summary of strength training types and the recipes required to produce the desired effect.[1]

Anatomical adaptation builds base strength and prepares the foundation for more intense and load-bearing exercises that lie ahead. The training load is not high, and the focus of these sessions is not to build muscle, but instead, to stimulate the nervous response in the brain and promote correct use and activation of existing muscles. Among other things, to "turn on" and strengthen small stabilizing muscles that are often inactive due to poor posture or

1   Adapted from the book *Periodization Training for Sports* by Tudor Bompa and Carlo Buzzichelli

lifestyle habits. This helps to optimize how the body moves and results in overall strength gains and prevents injuries.

- Training session examples: circuit strength training (not timed), Pilates, Yoga, functional strength training

Hypertrophy increases muscle size through growth of myofibrils (rod-like units of muscle fibers) in muscle tissue. While this kind of training does result in significant strength gains, the process is very taxing on the body due to the use of large weights and muscle failure. As a result, it requires a very long recovery time and impairs aerobic training that most athletes need to improve their athletic performance. Hypertrophy training is best used by athletes whose sport performance depends on larger size (i.e., shot putters, discus throwers).

- Training session examples: traditional weight training targeting muscle fatigue.

Maximum strength training achieves two things: it develops neurological pathways and promotes the growth of mitochondria in glycolytic muscle tissue. This improves muscle economy and maximizes the force that athletes can produce. In a way, it's similar to Zone 5 training. This type of training is what produces the biggest effect: an increase in the absolute force results in more powerful sport-specific movements and improved performance. However, athletes must give the muscles enough time to rest (3–5min between repeats) to regenerate their ATP/CP energy system. The purpose is not to fatigue muscles, but instead to be able to repeat the same maximum output again and again.

- Training session examples: maximum load training, explosive strength training.

Power development translates the ability to produce maximum output into muscular endurance and movement quality. In particular, athletes improve their ability to apply strength effectively in their respective sport by using short and explosive repeats (i.e., medicine ball throws), as well as maintaining high output for a longer period of time by overcoming resistance (i.e., bench press performed at fast speed). On a longer end (1–4 minutes), this is similar to VO_2max training and provides the same cardiovascular benefits.

- Training session examples: timed circuit strength training (i.e., boot-camp), Tabata workout, Calisthenics training, throws.

EXERCISE: REVIEW YOUR TRAINING INTENSITY

How aware are you of your training efforts? Training intensity is usually the reason why athletes experience training plateaus. They either do too much too soon and end up fatigued or don't challenge their bodies enough and miss out on the super-compensation effect. The key to progress is correct timing and making sure that the body is in the optimal condition to perform and process the training load.

For this exercise, I ask you to review the intensity you are training in. Calculate your training zones and analyze how your current and past aerobic training fits with those. Based on what you learned in this chapter, what effect do you think your efforts trigger? What effect are you looking for and are you looking for any particular one at all? Do the same for your strength training; what loads, velocity and rest intervals do you use in training and which training type do they correlate to?

You can use the heart rate zone calculator on my blog to help you determine the zones. Go to https://theathleteblog.com/heart-rate-zone-calculator/ and input your maximum and resting heart rates there.

Going forward, I challenge you to pay attention to which zone you are exercising in or what type of strength training you are doing. Think strategically and focus on the effect that the exercise triggers for your body. This will help to bring quality to the process, make it more effective, and help you to break through the training plateau.

PEAK IS A STEPPING STONE

A common notion being passed around is that competitive sport is detrimental to long-term health. Intense or prolonged exercise is seen as dangerous and people who engage in it will inevitably suffer from the consequences when they reach senior years. Endurance athletes in particular get bad rap because they tend to grind through the year and accumulate fatigue in pursuit of more miles. While concerns for health and vitality are always valid, especially given how many people approach fitness from a fanatic perspective, they can also be used as an excuse not to be more serious about taking up physical exercise… especially by people who don't know all the details. I noticed that such remarks, ironically, often come from people who either have already experienced burnout or haven't exercised in a structured manner themselves (or at all). For them, even a 3-hour training week (30 minutes of exercise six days a week) is already brutal.

There are people like Mariko Yugeta, a Japanese woman who at 62 years of age ran a 2:52:13 marathon, improving her own world record in the 60+ age group by more than four minutes. A middle-distance runner in high school, she didn't pick up serious marathon training until she was 41 and a mother of four kids. While according to the notion that extensive running should have caused her major health issues, she keeps improving and adding more volume year after year. And she's not alone. Ed Whitlock from Canada has been a lifelong distance runner and at 85 has completed a marathon in 3:56:34 (80+ age group record). Hiromu Inada from Japan who at 89 to this date is the oldest person who completed the Ironman triathlon. That list goes on and something is not adding up. Shouldn't all these people have heart, knee, hip and other health problems as a result of their lifelong high performance hobbies?

There are plenty of athletes who have engaged in high performance sports throughout their entire lives and as they reach senior years are still healthy and full of energy. Have these athletes discovered a secret recipe? Maybe they have, after all everyone is on a personal Hero's Journey to find their own elixir of life. However, as examples like Mariko show, athletes become resilient because they play the long game. They take time to develop aerobic base and strength to withstand such activities as a 30K run, a 5-hour bike ride, or even a 10-hour hiking day. They don't rush into training, but continue to develop a foundation that lets their fitness grow throughout the years and support new adventures.

Contrary to how it may seem, athletes do not live beyond the redline their entire lives. In fact, throughout the season, the majority of training is rather easy and doesn't push the limits on a daily basis. **That is because it's not possible to sustain peak fitness indefinitely.** Even elite athletes attain top condition for a few weeks only in preparation for a major competition. What they also do, however, is maintain a good base fitness throughout the year that allows them to "peak" for a specific event. Such maintenance is much less impactful on the body (but still very effective) and gives athletes the flexibility to choose when to deliver their best performance and capacity to become even better.

Sure, it is nice to be in the most optimal condition to deliver the best performance when it counts the most: whether that means qualifying for Boston, finishing an ultra-endurance race, or even trekking in the Himalayas. However, after the event is over there always comes the question: what now? Peak fitness is not the final destination. It is a stimulus for the body to go beyond what's comfortable and gradually adapt to a higher workload, so that next time it can go a little further. In a certain way, it's a stepping stone to an even bigger outcome. That's how training programs work: they challenge the athlete and then back off to let him or her recover before building again.

Rate of recovery is what makes all the difference and what all of the athlete's potential comes down to. There were many references to the importance of recovery for performance throughout the book and in this chapter, we will finally align the pieces of the puzzle.

GRADUAL ADAPTATION

Most athletes accept the fact that they need to train a great deal to become successful in their sport. **However, training with no particular plan in mind will be unlikely to yield great results.** Showing up a few times a week and repeating the same routine every time is what I call a "hobby sport." There is nothing wrong with that approach, as long as the individual is happy and uses exercise to unwind and enjoy themselves. However, if an athlete is looking to improve, a key element to success is an organized approach to training which helps to build fitness over time and optimize performance for target events (competitions or adventures) without becoming overstressed. Isn't this why you picked up this book in the first place?

The principle of gradual adaptation lies at the core of exercise physiology. According to it, an athlete can attain his or her desired fitness by applying relevant training stimuli at an appropriate rate. In other words, an athlete needs to provide just enough challenge to trigger the adaptation processes and then back off to let the body recover and super-compensate. Over time, these small incremental improvements total to a substantial shift in physical fitness and resilience. This is where self-awareness and being vigilant to the signals the body sends becomes vital.

One of the biggest mistakes I made as an athlete, and see among the people I coach, is not being honest about your level of current fitness. I used to overestimate how fit I was (and how fast I could go) and unintentionally trained harder than was required for optimal adaptation. As a result, my body was always under a constant training load and unable to adapt. It took me years to understand that the workload should be defined by my current fitness level and what the body is capable of adjusting to—not what I expected from it or what others are doing. Every athlete needs to start where they are and build the training load gradually from there.

A person who has recently started running does not need to follow the same schedule that elite runners do. A 30-minute jog three to five times per week is more than enough to begin building fitness. Trying to replicate a five or even ten-hour training week with intervals, two-hour long runs and strength training on top too soon will most likely just overload the body—or, worse, lead to injury.

Our bodies are capable of a lot more than we expect of them, but we need to listen to the signals they send to make intelligent decisions about when to back off. If we increase our training volume too much, the body will not be able to process it fully and some breakdown might occur—accumulated fatigue, burnout, or even an injury. What we want instead is to find the rate of change the body is comfortable with—the natural rate of training absorption. And for that the 10% rule is the best starting point.

According to the 10% rule, training volume should increase on average by no more than ten percent per week to produce sustainable adaptation.

You might have already noticed that the fitter you get, the more effort (both quality and quantity) is required to continue improving. So, to put your body on a growth trajectory, start with your current schedule and increase the total training volume by 10% the next week. Do the same next week. And the week after that. Soon what you felt was unreachable, becomes the usual as the body gradually adapts to a more challenging routine.

Let's take an example of Sophie to see how the 10% rule works in practice. She's been running for a few years and currently is comfortable covering 30 minutes three times per week (90 minutes in total). After chatting with some runner colleagues at work the other day, she has decided to increase her training volume in an effort to become a better and more resilient runner.

That can come from either of the three factors:

- **Duration:** The length of a training session, measured in time. If Sophie extends her runs from 30 minutes to an hour (what many athletes do), she will bump up her total training volume from 90 minutes to 180 minutes, a 100% change. A sharp increase like that will likely put a lot of stress on the legs, resulting in serious fatigue, pain or even injury. Instead, Sophie is better off adding 10% volume every week: 99 minutes, then 109, then 120. This way she will be able to almost double her running volume within two months and, in contrast to a sudden increase, will avoid the frustration of a setback and gain confidence and enthusiasm for success. If Sophie had developed pain or injury after doubling her volume within a week, after those same 2 months she probably would only be recovering from it.

- **Frequency**: The number of training sessions over a given period of time. An increase in the training frequency also affects the total volume and, therefore, should be considered under the 10% rule. If Sophie adds a fourth 30-minute run to her weekly schedule (another frequent mistake), it will increase the total volume by 33% to 120 minutes per week and will, therefore, result in more fatigue than necessary for sustainable adaptation. In order to include a fourth session, Sophie needs to shorten the other three and use the 10% rule to make sure the weekly volume increases gradually. So, if her total volume is 3x30=90 minutes, the next week can be 24+25+25+25=99 minutes (+10%). Then 109 and only then 120. With this approach, it is more likely that Sophie will adjust to the workload gradually and avoid overstressing the body.

- **Intensity:** The level of effort as measured by time in training zones. Besides gradual increase in training volume, it is important to pay attention to the proportion of moderate and high intensity in relation to it. For example, if Sophie decides to include a 20-minute tempo interval (Zone 3) into one of her training sessions, that will mean 22% of her weekly volume (90 minutes) will consist of moderate intensity, which is too much to begin with. It's far more sustainable to start with just 5 minutes of tempo effort (~5% of total volume) and apply the principle of gradual adaptation to increase it every week. Intensity is the exception to the 10% rule: on the lower end it can be increased faster, as long as the share of moderate and high intensity in the plan is low (under 10%).

Obviously, it is not possible to increase training volume indefinitely. So, to make sure the body gets adequate rest and is able to adapt, it is important to include so-called recovery weeks. A good practice is to reduce the training volume (typically by around 20%) for a week after every 3 weeks of build, and after that, pick up where you left off. Ideally, that downtime should cover all three factors: duration of the exercise, its frequency, and the length of intense intervals in it.

The principle of gradual adaptation should also be applied in situations when training has been skipped or paused. During a break, the body loses some fitness, and the usual workload becomes a little (or a lot) more challenging.

Here are a few tips on how to ease back into the training process safely and avoid putting excessive load on the body:

- **Skipping up to three days of training.** No big deal, treat it as recovery time. Feel free to resume the training process where you left off, but don't try to compensate for skipped sessions by doing more. Take the first day after such a break a bit easier.

- **Skipping one week.** Still not much fitness is lost. Athletes can catch up to their original training schedule and still maintain the same level of intensity. However, do reduce the training volume of the first week by 30% and take the first two days of it easy.

- **Skipping two or more weeks.** That is what I call an extended training break. If an athlete has not done any purposeful training for more than two weeks, he or she needs to re-evaluate the current fitness level and adjust the goal. It is best to come back to the level of training volume that's comfortable (often back to foundation) and start the process of building fitness from there.

TRAINING PERIODIZATION

As already discussed, an athlete needs to vary his or her training to become well-rounded and successful. However, it's not productive to try to improve everything at once. Nor is it possible, really. Different attributes often require almost opposite workouts to improve. Mitochondria (endurance gains) respond well to long easy sessions and short bursts of speed without exhaustion. Myofibrils (strength and size gains), on the other hand, grow the most in response to anaerobic training and fatigue.

When training for a race, many athletes try to jump straight into high intensity, thinking they need speedwork, intervals, tempo efforts; that these are what will make them faster. The problem with this reasoning is that if high intensity intervals are added when the aerobic capacity is small, the body cannot tolerate much of a training load and, therefore, improvements are quite limited. Also, it's not a good idea to put the body through a maximum load if the athlete has very tight and inflexible muscles—that's a recipe for injury. On the other hand, if that same athlete starts by making their muscles mobile and strong and in the meantime build aerobic capacity, he or she will be surprised at what kind of speed the body can sustain, even before formal speed training.

To make sure athletes are training effectively, they need to start easy and make gradual and timely changes to their training process. This approach is called **training periodization**. It includes splitting the process into different phases to focus on a particular attribute (i.e., flexibility, strength, endurance, speed, coordination). Each phase will include different types of training and have a specific recipe (intensity, volume, rest intervals) to challenge the body in a certain way. The goal of such periodization is to give an athlete the best possible chance of peak performance at a desired time. And all of it starts with a plan.

> *Consistent results are like a German vacation—they require a proper plan, preferably half a year in advance.*

Many athletes think of and plan their training from the perspective of days and weeks. '*What should I do during this particular session? How much time should I train this week?*' However, in order to maximize training effectiveness, we need to consider a longer perspective.

There's a lot of turbulence from day to day (i.e., fatigue, stress, missed workouts) and every individual session may not be reflective of the athlete's actual condition.

This is why the key to peaking is to plan long term. Not in days or weeks (known as microcycles), but instead in longer periods of several months or even years (known as meso- and macrocycles). Create a training plan by counting backwards from the moment you wish to deliver peak performance and split the time into phases to focus on one particular attribute at a time.

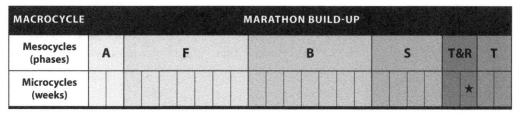

★ = Race, A = Adaptation, F = Foundation, B = Build-up,
S = Simulation, T&R = Taper and Race, T = Transition.

Figure X.X. Example of a 24–week periodized training process for a marathon runner.

In order to prepare for the race, we cannot repeat the same workouts all over again. There is a certain sequence in building fitness that makes the process effective. Start by improving your foundation by building strength and aerobic capacity with easy exercise. From there, proceed to add more volume and intensity to grow endurance and translate absolute strength into powerful sport-specific movements. Finally, focus on particular demands of a race (i.e., terrain, distance, intensity) to reach peak condition before tapering off. Ideally, every phase will add new training methods and incorporate some of the exercises and training sessions from the previous one, which will create a highly effective, yet healthy schedule.

Top athletes plan their seasons using the same pattern. They start with a training camp that focuses on long easy workouts and plenty of strength training. This is what brings them "back in shape." After that, depending on the race distance, they include moderate and high intensity to work on sport-specific strength and endurance. A few months out from the race, they increase intensity a little more to challenge the body a little more before tapering off for the competition.

The training load builds in the form of a wave. When an athlete prepares the body for the work ahead (adaptation phase), there is very little increase in the overall load. It starts to change during the foundation phase as workouts grow longer and some intensity is added via explosive strength training and short speed pick-ups.

During the build phase, training load starts to grow significantly because athletes add more moderate and high-intensity training into their schedule. Closer to race day, athletes increase intensity or duration further to provide stimulus for the body to "peak" (simulation phase) and reduce it in the following weeks to let the body reach optimal condition for the race (taper). After the race is completed, athletes take a few weeks to unwind (transition) and start preparing for the next adventure in the same way. Even though some fitness is lost during the last phase, it is required to give the body time to rest, recover and calm the nervous system down after months of training.

Throughout the years, an athlete goes through the same process many times. He or she builds, peaks, recovers, and then starts to build again. Each time from a bigger base, which allows them to peak even higher. Which is why building fitness is a multi-year process.

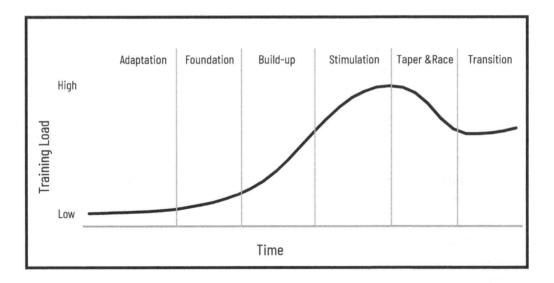

Development of the training load throughout different phases of a program.

Even though the load will gradually increase as the training progresses, depending on the phase the share of moderate and high intensity in the plan will vary. That is because intense training generates a lot of fatigue, and the body needs to be resilient enough to process it and train again shortly. A good rule of thumb is to make sure low intensity exercise (Zones 1 and 2) forms at least 80% of the training plan to give the body ample time to recover. This is known as

80/20 training. Some deviations from that rule are possible, so it is best to apply it to a longer time frame, several months or half a year. For instance, in the beginning of the training cycle, low intensity exercise might make up as much as 95% of the total volume (close to 100% in adaptation), whereas closer to the goal race in peak phase it can drop to 70%.

ADAPTATION

Most of the injuries occur as a result of imbalances in the body that develop throughout the years (i.e., due to sedentary lifestyle, inefficient form, past injuries). The first few weeks of the training plan is an opportunity to relieve tight muscles, improve range of motion, and build strength in supportive muscles as athletes ease into structured training. Doing so helps you to reduce and prevent pain, as well as make sure your body is well-balanced and can withstand pressure from longer and more intense training sessions that will follow.

ADAPTATION PHASE	
Purpose	Prepare the body for the intense training process ahead. In particular, align the body to prevent injuries throughout the training process
Duration	More experienced athletes—2 weeks Less experienced athletes—up to 6 weeks
Goals	Relieve muscle tension and improve range of motion Correct muscle imbalances Develop base strength
Aerobic Training Focus	Low intensity (Zones 1 + 2)—almost 100% of the total volume Low impact frequent and/or prolonged exercise (i.e., easy cycling, jogging).
	Moderate intensity (Zone 3)—minimum
	High intensity (Zones 4 + 5)—less than 5% of the total volume Optional: short and controlled hard accelerations (up to 30sec pick-ups to Zones 4 + 5 with ~1:4 work-to-rest ratio) for neuromuscular stimulation
Strength and Mobility Focus	Dynamic and deep (40+ seconds) stretches Mobility, core and balance exercises Bodyweight strength training (6–9 exercises, 10–20 repetition sets with little rest)

Overview of the adaptation phase in the training lifecycle.

The purpose of the adaptation phase is not to build power or endurance, but rather to get muscles used to exercising after a training break. Strength training is key and should be focused on slow and controlled execution, not on completing as many repetitions as possible. Besides growing base strength, this will also instill correct movement patterns that will optimize the body and help to prevent injuries.

The best approach to include such training is to focus on bodyweight exercises. These are usually compound movements that engage a lot of muscle fibers across the whole body—from prime movers to "stabilizers." In addition to that, the movements improve mobility and range of motion. Athletes should choose a training load so that they can complete exercises with little or no rest in between, which will ensure even the smallest stabilizing muscles are engaged.

As athletes begin structured training, they don't need much volume to see progress. A typical training session in this phase can last anywhere from 20–30 minutes to 1.5 hours. Besides base strength, the goal is to get into the habit of exercising frequently and moving every part of the body through a full range of motion. Since the intensity of such training is low, recovery is quick, and athletes can do a form of exercise every day.

MON	TUE	WED	THU	FRI	SAT	SUN
Active rest	**Aerobic** Z2 followed by **Strength** Body-weight	**Aerobic** Z2 followed by **Core** 10 min	Active rest	**Aerobic** Z2 followed by **Core** 10 min	**Strength** Body-weight	**Cross-training** i.e., hiking

Sample adaptation weekly plan for a runner.

FOUNDATION

Also known as "early base," the foundation phase focuses on building the initial fitness that athletes will carry through the season. In particular, the aerobic base that athletes develop during these months will make the body more efficient and speed up recovery time (thanks to the number of mitochondria that are built during prolonged training). It is an important stepping stone that makes athletes fatigue slower, tolerate more intensity later in the season (where it actually matters), and see more improvement. One doesn't need years to build that foundation. A couple of months of focused low intensity training will already provide a significant fitness boost.

Besides consistency that comes from the previous phase, one key habit that athletes should develop at this point is listening to the body and managing stress (both physical and mental). This includes getting consistent restful sleep, eating foods that nourish the body, meditation, and journaling (tracking workouts and noting down how the body feels before and after). The intensity of the training will only grow throughout the season, so it's important to learn to recognize the signals that the body sends and make timely adjustments to prevent burnout or overtraining.

FOUNDATION PHASE	
Purpose	Create foundation for intense sessions in the next phases. Improve aerobic capabilities. Prepare muscles and ligaments for the workload ahead
Duration	30–35% of the total plan
Goals	Develop aerobic base and power Strengthen muscles and ligaments Build absolute (maximum) strength
Aerobic Training Focus	Low intensity (Zones 1 + 2)—around 90% of the total volume Prolonged easy exercise (1+ hours for Zone 2 and 2+ hours for Zone 1)
	Moderate intensity (Zone 3)—up to 10% of the total volume Short strength-focused moderate intervals (i.e., uphill running, low-cadence cycling, work against resistance) Long tempo efforts (10–30 minutes)
	High intensity (Zones 4 + 5)—less than 5% of the total volume Short and controlled hard accelerations (up to 30sec pick-ups to Zones 4–5 with ~1:4 work-to-rest ratio) for neuromuscular stimulation
Strength and Mobility Focus	Mobility, core and balance exercises Maximum load training (3–5 prime mover exercises, 1–4 repetition sets with long rest)

Overview of the foundation phase in the training lifecycle.

A solid aerobic foundation takes time to build and is subject to previous training, experience in sport, current level of fitness, and dedication. Typically, significant results (lower heart rate or faster pace on easy runs) can be seen after around 15–20 hours of consistent aerobic work. Gathering that minimum volume can take months, so if you have an opportunity, this is a great time to plan a training camp for yourself to grow the aerobic base quicker (even if it is as short as an extended weekend). It is very beneficial to add a strength component to this aerobic development. When an athlete overcomes additional resistance (i.e., during trail running or low cadence cycling), he or she recruits more muscle fibers and promotes mitochondria growth in them, which translates to better muscle efficiency.

At this point of the program, the global stress is rather low, even though more volume and moderate intensity is added to grow aerobic base and strength. As a result, an athlete's recovery is quick and allows for more focused strength and conditioning sessions. After preparing the muscles and joints with initial adaptations, athletes can proceed to a more explosive work that will help to develop the maximum force the body can produce. This is done by lifting heavy loads or doing intense exercise for a very short period of time (less than 10 seconds) and a very long rest interval to avoid muscle exhaustion. This approach allows the athlete to repeat the effort many times, and besides improving absolute strength, also results in additional endurance gains.

MON	TUE	WED	THU	FRI	SAT	SUN
Active rest	**Run** Z2, incl. 4x20sec strides in Z4 followed by **Strength** Maximum load	**Cross-training** i.e., cycling, swimming followed by **Core** 10 min	**Run** Z2, incl. Z3 tempo intervals	**Strength** Maximum load	**Run** Z2, incl. 4x20sec strides in Z4 followed by **Core** 10 min	**Run** Long Z2 on hilly terrain

Sample foundation weekly plan for a runner.

BUILD-UP

The build-up phase is the extension of the base phase (sometimes called "late base") and is an important period for any athlete. The purpose of it is to build efficiency by blending the aerobic base, absolute strength and correct movement patterns that were developed in earlier phases into one balanced mechanism. Athletes use this phase to add specificity to their training. Besides growing more muscular endurance and improving anaerobic fitness, they also work on conditioning the muscle groups that are more specific to the sport to make them as powerful as possible.

Building on the habit of listening to the body, it is important to remember that mental strength is as important as physical strength. This phase of the season is a great time to develop resilience by training in hard conditions (rain, wind) and practicing self-regulating (having the courage to take a session easy when the body is under-recovered).

BUILD-UP PHASE	
Purpose	Develop race-specific speed and endurance
Duration	30–35% of the total plan
Goals	Develop aerobic capacity Develop anaerobic capacity (for shorter races) Develop power Build sport-specific strength
Aerobic Training Focus	Low intensity (Zones 1 + 2)—80% of the total volume • Short recovery sessions (30–40 minutes) • Prolonged easy exercise (1+ hours)
	Moderate intensity (Zone 3)—up to 10% of the total volume • Long tempo efforts (10–30 minutes) • Short tempo efforts (<10 minutes) as part of an easy long session
	High intensity (Zones 4 + 5)—up to 10% of the total volume • Medium-length "sweet spot" intervals (6–12 minutes repeats in low-/mid-Zone 4 with ~1:0,3–0,5 work-to-rest ratio) • Short threshold/VO_2max intervals (2–5 minutes repeats in high-Zone 4/low-Zone 5 with ~1:0,5–1 work-to-rest ratio) • Short speed intervals (up to 40sec repeats at close to maximum intensity with 1:3–6 work-to rest ratio) • Short and controlled hard accelerations (up to 30sec pick-ups to Zone 4–5 with ~1:4 work-to-rest ratio) for neuromuscular stimulation

BUILD-UP PHASE	
Strength and Mobility Focus	Mobility, core and balance exercises Muscular endurance training (1–4 minutes repeats with short rest) Functional strength and conditioning (3–6 explosive repetitions with short rest)

Overview of the build-up phase in the training lifecycle.

The demands of every sport are different and physical attributes that allow an athlete to throw a javelin well will not 100% translate into swimming strength or endurance. Even though the same muscle groups might be involved to perform the movements (i.e., back, shoulders, triceps, core), the biomechanics of every sport and the force application is different. Which is why after training general fitness in the previous phases, athletes need to develop anaerobic capabilities, as well as condition themselves. This can be accomplished through practicing sport-specific movements to make them more powerful.

During the build-up phase, the duration of aerobic sessions is kept constant (for short-distance events it may even decrease) and the training load increases on account of intensity. In particular, threshold repeats (hard Zone 4 intervals) are introduced to improve power and muscular endurance. These types of sessions improve "cruising" speed, as well as train the anaerobic energy system to tolerate buildup of lactate better, which helps both long-distance and short-distance athletes. On top of that in this phase, moderate intervals can be incorporated into longer training sessions to improve aerobic capacity.

Strength training takes a more specialized form as well. More intensity is added by increasing the speed of execution and adding conditioning drills (eccentric sport-specific movements), which builds both resistance to fatigue, functional strength, and greater efficiency. In particular, many athletes in this phase will benefit from the so-called plyometric exercises: fast and explosive movements in various directions repeated in quick succession. Jumping is a great example as it is a short but powerful effort that helps to condition muscles and joints. In fact, they say the day you stop jumping is the day you start ageing. However, since plyometric movements are very taxing, the number of exercises and repetitions should be kept low.

MON	TUE	WED	THU	FRI	SAT	SUN
Active rest	**Run** Z4 repeats followed by **Strength** Functional	**Run** Z1 followed by **Core** 10 min	**Cross-training** i.e., cycling, swimming	**Run** Z2, incl. Z3 tempo intervals followed by **Strength** Functional	**Run** Z2, incl. 4x20sec strides in Z4 followed by **Core** 10 min	**Run** Long Z2

Sample build-up weekly plan for a runner.

RACE-SPECIFIC

The several weeks leading into the race is the hardest block of training. It is dedicated to race-specific preparation and focuses on simulating the stresses the athlete will experience during the race. This is a very sensitive period as the workload reaches its peak and due to a lot of cortisol produced, white blood cells are not able to fight infections as effectively. As a result, the body's immune system is very weakened and it is very easy to end up sick, injured or overtrained and compromise the whole training process. Be careful and continue to stick to the 10% rule to make sure the body does not experience sudden changes in training volume. The body is only able to tolerate high intensity to a certain extent and for a limited period of time, which is why this kind of training comes at the very end. For longer events, the peak week of training typically takes place 4–5 weeks out from the race; for shorter races, it's 2 weeks.

The race-specific phase also serves as a rehearsal for the race. Besides tailoring the duration and intensity of training to get the body used to race pace, athletes can also simulate race situations and practice other important elements: terrain (i.e., climbs), race starts, nutrition, transition skills. This is a great opportunity to practice visualization technique (introduced in Chapter 6) and mentally prepare for how the race can unfold. Something always goes wrong on race day, which is why it is important to be prepared not only physically, but mentally. What does your warmup routine for the race look like? How will you pace yourself during a marathon? What would you do if you got a punctured tire in the middle of the bike leg during a triathlon? What would you do if your goggles snapped in the first minutes of the swim?

Purpose	Simulate demands of a race—both physiological and tactical
Duration	4–8 weeks (or up to 20% of the total plan)
Goals	Practice "race pace" and nutrition Simulate race conditions (weather, terrain, altitude, etc.) Create environment that helps to maximize key sessions (focus on recovery)
Aerobic Training Focus	Low intensity (Zones 1 + 2)—no less than 70% of the total volume • Short recovery sessions (30–40 minutes) • Prolonged easy exercise (1+ hours)
	Moderate intensity (Zone 3)—up to 20% (depending on the race) • Race pace practice efforts (for races over 2 hours in duration)—standalone intervals or incorporated in longer sessions • Short tempo efforts (<10 minutes) to supplement threshold sessions • Long tempo efforts (10–30 minutes)
	High intensity (Zones 4 + 5)—up to 20% (depending on the race) • Medium-length "sweet spot" intervals (6–12 minutes repeats in low-/mid-Zone 4 with ~1:0,3–0,5 work-to-rest ratio) as part of race pace practice (up to 20 minutes of total "work") • Short threshold/VO$_2$max intervals (2–5 minutes repeats in high-Zone 4/low-Zone 5 with ~1:0,5–1 work-to-rest ratio) • For short duration races: Short speed intervals (up to 40sec repeats at close to maximum intensity with 1:3–6 work-to rest ratio) • Short and controlled hard accelerations (up to 30sec pick-ups to Zone 4–5 with ~1:4 work-to-rest ratio) for neuromuscular stimulation
Strength and Mobility Focus	Mobility, core and balance exercises Functional strength and conditioning (3–6 explosive repetitions with short rest)

Overview of the race-specific phase in the training lifecycle.

In this phase, training is similar to the build phase, but there is more of it and it's more intense. The idea is to train at and slightly above race effort to get the body used to it and make it feel easier come race day. Generally, a hard training day (i.e., long session with intervals or high intensity intervals) should be followed by two or even three easy or recovery days (Zones 1 and 2) to let the body fully recover. As much as it is tempting to go harder when fitness is reaching its peak, it is important to take those easy days really easy to make sure the body has the capacity to put quality effort in on key days. Both volume and intensity on key days should simulate (but not 100% replicate) what an athlete would experience in a race.

While the focus of the race-specific phase is on the sport-specific activities, athletes will benefit from maintaining a strength training routine. However, it should focus on preventing the loss of strength only in order to not take away the energy from key race preparation. For that, short explosive sport-specific movements are the best option.

MON	TUE	WED	THU	FRI	SAT	SUN
Active rest	**Run** Z4 repeats followed by **Core** 10 min	**Run** Z1	**Run** Z2, incl. Z3 tempo intervals followed by **Strength** Explosive/ Functional	**Cross- training** i.e., cycling, swimming	**Run** Z2, incl. 4x20sec strides in Z4 followed by **Core** 10 min	**Run** Long Z2, incl. Marathon effort

Sample race-specific weekly plan for a marathon runner in the leadup to the goal race.

TAPER

Taper is the long-awaited period of complete recovery before the race. It's that part of the training plan where sessions are getting shorter, energy and mood improves, and athletes are feeling stronger than they have ever been. The goal of this phase is to carefully balance training volume, intensity, recovery, and nutrition, so that accumulated fatigue dissipates while the body is still in the supercompensation state. Doing so will allow an athlete to achieve the best condition within a relatively narrow window—the peak.

Race week in particular can feel a little weird, because there is less training than usual. To avoid filling free time with more training, it is a good idea to spend extra time focusing on organizational things and planning race logistics. Consider what time to wake up and what to eat for breakfast. What clothes to pack for the race and for the warmup. Decide when to leave for the start, and so on. Having a plan for race day removes a lot of stress and can help to focus better on delivering the best performance.

TAPER PHASE	
Purpose	Achieve top condition for the race.
Duration	Shorter races—1 week Longer races—up to 3 weeks
Goals	Reach peak fitness by gradually reducing volume and maintaining intensity Maintain optimal mental state by staying calm and not doubting yourself (or your coach)
Aerobic Training Focus	Low intensity (Zones 1 + 2)—no less than 90% of the total volume • Short recovery sessions (30–40 minutes) • Prolonged easy exercise (1+ hours)
	Moderate intensity (Zone 3)—5–10% (depending on the race) • Short race pace practice efforts (for races over 2 hours in duration)—standalone intervals or incorporated in longer sessions
	High intensity (Zones 4 + 5)—5–10% (depending on the race) • Short threshold/VO_2max intervals (2–5 minutes repeats in high-Zone 4/low-Zone 5 with ~1:0,5–1 work-to-rest ratio) • Short race pace practice efforts (organized in a 'fartlek' session, preferably with 1:1 work-to-rest ratio) • Short and controlled hard accelerations (up to 30sec pick-ups to Zone 4–5 with ~1:4 work-to-rest ratio) for neuromuscular stimulation
Strength and Mobility Focus	Mobility, core and balance exercises Functional strength and conditioning (3–6 explosive repetitions with short rest)

Overview of the taper phase in the training lifecycle.

They say you cannot build more fitness during the last week, but you can sacrifice what you've gained by training too much. The best way to achieve the best condition for the race is to progressively decrease the duration of sessions every week. Cut the total time by 30% in the first week of the taper and by another 50% during race week (or by 30–30–50 if it's a longer taper). Such a reduction in training duration, does not mean a reduction in intensity. Decreasing both can be detrimental to performance, so it is important to maintain regular intensity up to a few days out from a race. In particular, shorter intervals at or above race pace will help to sustain muscle economy and prevent loss of fitness.

> *It's natural to be curious and to test yourself with harder or longer efforts during sessions, don't do that. Stick to the training plan and have faith in it. Save that "extra" for the race.*

During taper phase, strength training has a supportive role only. Athletes can use sport-specific movements to activate the relevant muscles but should avoid exhausting the body.

MON	TUE	WED	THU	FRI	SAT	SUN
Active rest	**Run** fartlek—short Z4 repeats followed by **Strength** Functional	**Run** Z1 followed by **Core** 10 min	**Cross-training** i.e., cycling, swimming	**Run** Z2, incl. Z3 tempo intervals followed by **Strength** Functional	**Run easy** Z2, incl. 4x20sec strides in Z4 followed by **Core** 10 min	**Run** Long Z2, incl. Marathon effort
Active rest	**Run** fartlek—short Z4 repeats	**Cross-training** i.e., Z1 cycling, swimming	**Run (short)** Z2, incl. 4x20sec strides in Z4	Active rest	**Run (short)** Z2, incl. 4x20sec strides in Z4	**RACE**

Sample 2-week taper plan for a marathon runner.

TRANSITION

As much as some of us would like to, we cannot endlessly go beyond our comfort zone and live in the go-go-go mode. At some point, the body will run out of reserves and will force the athlete to rest—be it via overtraining, injury, or illness. Scheduling training breaks is a healthy practice that offsets the effects of a grueling training schedule and helps to keep the athletes healthy. In fact, it is one of the most important factors that ensures longevity in any sport.

Some of the athletes do not have one single race on the agenda. Instead, the racing schedule contains many smaller races (or events) every few weeks. That usually happens for shorter distance events (i.e., athletics, swimming, kayaking) or team competitions (i.e., volleyball, soccer). If that is the case, athletes can have a short break after the competition (a few days to a week) and resume training in the build phase. From there, they should proceed again to the race-specific phase, peak and taper for the next competition.

Athletes who don't have a structured approach to training often don't take the time to fully recover after the season (or a race). Instead, they try to preserve the fitness they worked hard to build by training through the year and not taking time off. While, indeed, some fitness will be lost during such a transition phase, a break from training is a necessary compromise that allows the body to fully recover and absorb the training load. If athletes return from a training break gradually (by using a periodized approach), then the period of rest will set the athlete up for an even better result in the next season.

A peak is just a stepping stone to an even bigger outcome next time.

Transition starts after the key (or last) race of the season and its goal is to let the body heal and recover from the long-term pressure it was operating under. Heal any injuries or muscle damage, replenish energy and vitamin/mineral reserves and, more importantly, recharge the nervous system and willpower.

It's good practice to take a couple of weeks completely off after every season and use this time to invest in yourself. Reconnect with hobbies, spend more time with family and friends, catch up on all the activities you have been missing out on. This doesn't necessarily mean doing nothing; many athletes stay active during that time but are not doing any purposeful training. It's a great opportunity to put all that fitness you have built to good use: do a form of cross-training or enjoy other activities you had no time for (like surfing or team sports).

The end of the season can be a very uninspiring time as all of the races or adventures are far in the future. The transition period can help to detach from training and return with more structure and focus. Take some time to reflect on what worked, what didn't, and what were the limiting factors during the entire preparation phase. Take 1–2 of the most significant ones and create a plan on how to fix those during the next few months. Such productive time off ensures that athletes will resume training with more quality and use the time until the active season starts to improve the foundation and address any weaknesses or imbalances.

EXERCISE: ORGANIZE YOUR TRAINING

One of the best ways to become a resilient athlete and ensure training is consistent is to have a periodized training plan. An athlete doesn't need to spend all of their free time on training to get good results. Nor does he or she need to sacrifice health to be competitive. In this chapter, I shared the principles that can help you develop a healthy training schedule that is effective, yet sustainable and ensures you continue improving as the training progresses throughout the years. Now it's time for you to apply that knowledge.

In this exercise, I ask you to look at your training as a coach, not as an athlete. Take out your training diary or create a spreadsheet. You will be creating a season plan for yourself—one that will ensure that you will reach a new peak. Use the guidelines shared in this part of the book to complete the three-step process below:

1. **Set a goal.** Be honest with yourself and determine your weak areas (i.e., strength, endurance, speed, form, agility). Set a priority for the season—what area you wish to improve—and write down the type of training that will help you achieve that. Is it developing an aerobic base? Increasing maximum force? Or something else?

2. **Split into phases.** Define the goal race or the adventure of the season where you want to show up at your absolute best. Count backwards from that date and split the time into relevant phases (adaptation, foundation and so on) to focus on one specific fitness attribute at a time. Give yourself time and make sure you spend plenty of it on building a solid

foundation. Try to also think how the season might unfold: when would you have more time to train, which races or travels you have in mind and so on.

3.   **Sort out the details.** Split the phases further into weeks and add specific training sessions you intend to complete. Vary the type of training depending on the phase. Make sure the plan is adapted to your lifestyle, takes the current fitness level into account and is balanced in low, moderate and high intensity (use the guidelines shared in this chapter). There is no point in having a plan which you cannot follow. Start with the training volume that you are currently comfortable with and increase it gradually (follow the 10% rule).

GO FAST OR GO FAR?

njuries suck. Being forced to pause training or even slow down an entire lifestyle until they heal can be devastating. Nor is it particularly enjoyable to have a nagging discomfort or ache somewhere. It is not exclusive to athletes; when a mild pain occurs, the response of the majority of people is to disregard it and organize life to avoid it instead of addressing the underlying problem. In fact, the older a person is, the higher the chance he or she has a certain muscular or joint ailment. A bad knee, an injured shoulder or the classic one, lower back pain. We tend not to think about injuries. Certainly not until they occur. Instead, we act as if we are invincible, asking the body to do more without taking care of it. *'Training is going great, which means I'm doing fine.'*

I had my fair share of injuries and noticed that all of them follow a similar pattern. There is almost always some muscle tightness that doesn't go away. Gradually, it grows into discomfort that stays even during training (or any other activity). With more workload, that discomfort gets painful or, even worse, an accident happens that forces the muscle or joint beyond its limited capability and shows us that we are not, in fact, bulletproof.

There was one particular incident that has taught me how disruptive a lack of forward thinking can be. Back when I ended my competitive kayaking career, I didn't stop training. My routine remained pretty consistent and included a few strength sessions paired with some indoor rowing and running every week. It was not as intense, but I felt like I was making good progress, especially on the muscle building front I've struggled with previously. That was until winter began.

During a trip to the mountains, I had a skiing accident where my boot mount came loose and I fell on my back, spraining my shoulder. Luckily, I didn't tear any of the ligaments or break any bones, but it was a significant sprain that healed painfully slowly. I couldn't run fast, couldn't lift heavy objects or do anything active for that matter. Any impact would send sharp shockwaves and cracking sensations right into my shoulder.

Even after six months the pain was still there. MRI scans showed I had some inflammation and a sports medicine surgeon explained that I seem to have developed a so-called shoulder impingement. In very simple terms, he explained to me that the shoulder blade and the upper-arm bone are positioned very close to each other and "rub" on the rotator cuff tendons that stabilize the shoulder. That irritates them thereby creating inflammation and pain. A small surgery would be necessary to investigate and, potentially, create more space in the joint. The surgery is called arthroscopy and is, apparently, a standard practice: cut it, fix it and an athlete is back into training mode within 6 weeks.

Something didn't feel right. Even though surgery seemed like an easy way to fix it, I wasn't a fan of the idea. How had I injured my shoulder so "irreversibly" with one single fall that it requires external intervention, while kids tumble daily as they learn to ski and still carry on? After all, the tendons were not torn, so shouldn't it be possible for them to heal on their own? I believed there was another way, so I went to get other opinions.

Finally, one orthopedic surgeon told me what I secretly wanted to hear: train more and train better. He explained to me that my shoulder joint was "misplaced" due to muscle imbalance. Tight chest muscles pulled it inward, while rotator cuff muscles were not strong enough to stabilize it back. Such a compromised position can create irritation and pain even without the skiing accident. In fact, had my shoulder been mobile and strong, I probably wouldn't even have the injury in the first place. But there was hope. I could use training not only to reverse that condition, but also prevent something like this from happening again. Among others, light exercises that rotate the shoulder internally and externally would help to put the joint back into the correct position as the stabilizing muscles get stronger. So, the more I trained, the less pain I would feel.

Unfortunately, my experience is not unique. Thousands of people (athletes or not) go through the same problem on a daily basis. **Due to lack of movement and stimulation muscles in certain areas of the body become tight, weak, and imbalanced, which creates nagging discomfort or pain.** Think about it, when we were kids, we were able to do anything and were so mobile that any fall would hardly hurt us. However, as we go through life, we tend to spend more time not moving (i.e., sitting or lying down), which sets up the stage for a potential injury.

Somehow when people are overweight, they generally understand that diet and exercise will reverse their condition. With joint pain it's different. There's typically no awareness of what to do, so when pain or discomfort occurs it's often ignored or linked to age or old injuries. As a result, many people postpone action until invasive surgery is the only way to go. But it doesn't have to be that way. Our body is very resilient and, in many cases, aches and discomforts can be reversed by taking care of the body and building it stronger. Not necessarily training to get better, but doing the regular maintenance, so to speak. It's not a stand-in for sports medicine but looking after the body in such a way can help it to relieve stress and stay ready to perform. It makes the training process sustainable, and, most importantly, it helps us to avoid the consequences that prevent us from living fully in the future.

MOBILITY

Every day, we are fed this notion that humans tend to lose some range of motion in their joints with age. It is a beautiful story to explain why so many people are struggling with injuries or are less active than they used to be. However, even though it sounds attractive and convincing, it's just a story. The world is filled with examples of people in their 70s maintaining the mobility that a typical 30-year-old could wish for and, more importantly, are living life fully. And don't forget about the yogis well in their 80s or even 90s who seem to be able to tie themselves in a knot.

In truth, subscribing to the notion that people lose mobility with age is nothing more than another limiting belief. **We lose it if we don't use it because it's a function of a lifestyle, not a predetermined setting.** Once we step into "the real world," and start our careers, we tend to spend extended periods of time sitting down (at the desk or elsewhere), which makes muscles across the body tight and weak. We don't run, jump, roll around or otherwise move in every direction as much as we did when we were kids, so we don't utilize the full range of motion that the body is capable of.

Without enough stimulus, some of the muscle mass atrophy (including stabilizing muscles) and, in an attempt to optimize itself, the body naturally shortens the range of motion which gradually becomes the "new norm." That is, until the moment we realize we can't reach our toes, touch our fingers behind our backs, extend our arms fully overhead or even stand up straight without discomfort.

There's more to the story. Tight muscles and limited range of motion impacts connective tissue that runs through our body and contributes to the formation of the so-called scar tissue: abnormal binding between muscles. Sometimes these bindings can compress and pinch nerves, causing inflammation and leading to injuries like strains and tears in various areas of the body.

All muscles and joints are connected across the body. Often what hurts is not where the problem is.

There are several areas in our body where people commonly feel discomfort: lower back, neck, knee, ankle, and shoulders, among others. Often it occurs as a result of a sedentary lifestyle, but athletes can experience pain and discomfort due to muscle overuse as well. The worst part is that the place that hurts is usually not where the underlying problem is. The body is a complex structure and when a certain area of it gets tight or overused the load is spread to the adjacent muscles and joints, which puts them under excess pressure.

For instance, when hip flexors and hamstrings get overloaded (due to fatigue or tightness), there is more load on the lower back to balance the body, which can result in pain. To take another example, tightness in hips and quads creates a limited range of motion in the lower body and puts more pressure on the knees to balance, which can also create pain. Every person's situation is unique, therefore the best way to prevent injuries is to ensure the overall body is mobile and aligned.

As painful and frustrating as it was, the shoulder injury I suffered from was, probably, the best thing that could happen in my athletic career. It made me slow down and learn how muscle imbalances develop, how they limit performance and why injury prevention is critical for an athlete. Structurally, the body doesn't get compromised in a day or even a week; it's almost always a series of small limitations that the body gradually adjusts to. It is not possible to reverse these changes overnight with a few stretches, but instead requires a structured approach to build a solid foundation for the years ahead. That approach consists of three parts: heal, release, and strengthen.

- **Heal.** Whenever there's pain or discomfort, it's important to let the body rest and try to take care of the issue itself. Once the inflammation has developed, it takes time for it to subside, and any additional physical activity can slow that process down. If you feel like something is off, reduce the workload, cross train to focus on other muscle groups, or better yet, take a break from training completely. A few days away from training can be just enough to relieve the discomfort and avoid overstressing the body. Often, athletes try to train through the pain in hopes that it shall pass on its own. Sometimes it does, but often it develops into a bigger issue and forces them to take a bigger break. Even experienced athletes who are good at recognizing good pain (i.e., soreness from a workout) and bad pain (a developing injury) can get overambitious about how far they can push themselves.

- **Release.** Tight muscles restrict movement, which ultimately leads to discomfort or pain. So, the next step is to return to the regular range of motion. Once the immediate pain has subsided, evaluate the situation. Localize the discomfort and determine what muscles caused it. This is the time to contact an orthopedic specialist, a physical therapist, or even a good masseur who will be able to tell which areas are restricted or tight, as well as help to relieve the pressure (i.e., with active release techniques or deep tissue massage). However, athletes can release a lot of tightness themselves with purposeful stretching and mobility work. Use deep stretching (slight discomfort, over 1 minute in duration) to release key areas and large muscle groups that most commonly get overused: hips, quads, chest, back. Additionally, move the joints (hips, knees, ankles, shoulders, elbows and wrists) through their full range of motion to mobilize them and improve the blood flow.

- **Strengthen.** The final step in the injury reversion process is to address the underlying problem: weakness in stabilizing muscles that causes poor alignment. It is not a quick process; it takes months (or even years) to lose the range of motion and functional strength, so patience and an organized approach is needed to build it back. Once you do, however, the pain will not return. The goal of such functional strength training is to re-introduce the full range of motion into daily life and exercise, as well as engage smaller supportive muscles that are often underdeveloped. This is achieved with core and rehabilitation exercises. There is minimum to no load in these, because stabilization muscles are much smaller than key muscle groups. The speed of execution is very slow and controlled. Swinging or rushing the movement will force stronger muscles to compensate and make the exercise useless. The focus is not to lift the heaviest weight possible but introduce a correct movement pattern.

Nagging issues might seem minor at first, but throughout the years we unintentionally use them to discount beliefs about our own capabilities. Remember the Circle of Life from

Chapter 3? Every small discomfort or ache we experience is like a small crack in the armor that affects what we focus on (pain vs. growth), our willingness to take action and our results or experiences that ultimately confirm or disprove the beliefs of what we are capable of.

It's like a self-fulfilling prophecy. A person who thinks he's incapable of something becomes incapable and a person who thinks he's old becomes old. People run marathons when they are 60, learn to surf at the age of 70 and even practice and teach yoga beyond the age of 80. Being mobile and injury-free allows us to retain the required strength to function well throughout life and, more importantly, have the confidence to enjoy what our bodies can do. **This is the key to living life to the fullest—we have no excuse.**

A lot of discomfort and chronic pain which we learned to live with over the years can be reversed with the right training protocol. Imagine that there are no restrictions on your fitness. No bad knees, shoulder pain or aching lower back. How full would your life be? What would you go on to experience?

CASE STUDY: REVERSE PAIN WITH MOBILITY

Eva is a 37-year-old small business owner and an avid traveler who has recently discovered an opportunity to explore new places by means of endurance challenges. She has already completed a few marathons and is looking to step into multisport with the half-Ironman triathlon on the agenda a few months from now.

Eva has been running 3–4 days per week for a few years and has never experienced a serious injury apart from some calf pain during her first year of training. So, as the weather warmed up, she increased her running volume in addition to indoor cycling and the occasional commute by bicycle. After a month or so, the outside of her knee started to hurt. It got so bad that she was able to run for no more than 10 minutes before the pain forced her to slow down to a walk. That was when she asked me for training advice.

What Eva suffered from is a condition commonly known to runners as Iliotibial Band (or IT Band) syndrome. Average recovery? Up to several months if left untreated. The combination of running, cycling and sitting at work has made her hips so tight that they started "pulling" the IT band, which resulted in knee pain. To address the situation, Eva took a week of very light training during which she focused on releasing tightness in the hips (with foam rolling) and gradually adding strengthening exercises: hip external and internal rotation, side leg raises and core work. Surprisingly, that solved the problem and the next week she didn't feel pain during her run.

While this is a miraculous example of recovery, it could have been prevented in the first place had only Eva included different movements into her training routine. She essentially worked in two dimensions only—legs moving forward or backward—and extra running volume only brought that issue to the surface. What Eva needed was to challenge the body in various ways (moving sideways, turning, rotating, etc.) to build strength in all areas of the body, not only in big muscle groups. Add a session of Yoga or Pilates once a week, do a form of mobility every morning or even as little as 5–10 minutes of core and stabilization exercises following a training session. It sounds simple but can prevent an athlete being forced to spend months in recovery from an injury.

Small stabilizing muscles (and core in particular) are responsible for keeping our body aligned and functioning effectively. That stability—among other things—improves performance, promotes good posture, and reduces the risk of many injuries. When muscles are underdeveloped (compared to other muscle groups or not used enough in daily life), the body is not able to align itself, which forces the body to compensate in a certain way often leading to overuse, muscle imbalance, discomfort or even pain.

WHAT IS PREHAB?

Being able to run fast, endure more, lift heavy or even live fully is largely dependent on the functional movement patterns that the body follows. An athlete with good form and alignment will be able to perform better (and longer), whereas poor form will not allow him or her to use the body's entire capacity, ultimately leading to premature fatigue. Besides that, restricted mobility and muscle imbalance are key indicators of an upcoming injury. When either of the athlete's sides (left vs. right or front vs. back) is significantly stronger, there is a high chance that pain will develop as a result of overuse.

Athletes are type A personalities and we always strive to achieve more. Performance in any of its interpretations is our passion. I am like that myself and see such a spark in every athlete I coach. However, it comes at a cost: slowing down does not come easy to us and in such a mindset it's very common to lose touch with oneself. Which is why even though it seems minor, it is necessary to take time and address any structural issues or inefficiencies. A small crack in the foundation can bring the entire house down and a small discomfort can amplify into pain and injury if not treated. I experienced what physical therapists mean when they joke about how every athlete either has been injured or will be injured. Before my shoulder injury, I didn't know how debilitating being on the sidelines is and thought I was bulletproof. Injury and pain that lasted for nearly 2 years made me become more careful about how I treat my body.

Athletes who have gone through a long rehabilitation process look at performance differently. They value alignment and functional strength and aim to ensure that the body operates as effectively as possible. **They call it prehab: proactively engaging in certain activities to compensate for the repetitive movements and stresses of regular training (or life, for that matter).** Correcting dysfunctions, restoring biomechanics, and optimizing movements. In other words, preventing injuries before they happen and making the body more resilient in the long term. Improved performance comes as a bonus. The idea behind is the same as rehabilitation, only prehabilitation (or prehab) takes place before something has gone wrong.

The difference between rehab and prehab is that the former is forced following an injury and the latter is proactive and preventative.

Prehab is not limited to a few stretches and exercises here and there, but rather a systemic approach. In a way, it also requires a change in the mindset which, by this point in the book, you are starting to develop.

EFFECTIVE WARM-UP

If you care about the body and don't want it to break down, you need to prepare it for the workload before a training practice or generally in the morning. And not just by "shaking the legs" a bit and doing a few arm swings—a proper warmup is much more than that.

Warmer muscles work more effectively than cold ones, as the blood travels faster and delivers oxygen more effectively. Besides getting muscles warm, a warmup also improves the range of motion and helps to remove any tightness, which makes movements more powerful and efficient. The whole process should include only dynamic movements. Static stretching and/or stretching "cold" muscles only puts additional pressure on them and greatly increases the risk of strains and other injuries.

LOWER BODY	TORSO	UPPER BODY
Ankle circles	Torso circles	Neck circles
Knee circles	Jumping oblique twists	Shoulder circles
Waist circles	Cat-cow flow	Wrist/palm circles
Leg swings (linear and lateral)	Forward-backward bends	Elbow twists
Hip rotation	Side bends	Arm circles
Downward dog to lunge flow	Bent-over windmills	German arm swings
Toy soldiers	Child's pose to cobra pose flow	Diagonal arm swings

Basic warmup exercises.

Low intensity and recovery sessions do not require much warm up—ten minutes of dynamic stretches and basic exercises is generally enough to loosen up stiff muscles. However, during higher intensity sessions the demands are higher, and the risk of injury is greater, therefore in addition to dynamic stretching athletes should also activate the muscles that will take the most load during the session, as well as smaller stabilizing muscles which help to maintain good and efficient form. Besides preventing injuries, this habit sets the body up for better performance by prolonging time to fatigue and improving power/speed.

A proper warmup typically takes 10–20 minutes for a training session (depending on intensity) and around 45 minutes for a race.

It consists of the following three parts:

- **Basic warmup exercises and dynamic stretches** to release muscle tightness. During the movement, take your muscles through a normal range of motion to the point of light tension and back. Twisting, turning, and moving the limbs in different directions extends their range of motion and speeds up the blood flow. The best results are achieved when athletes start with the biggest muscle groups and work their way to the smallest ones.

- **Easy aerobic activity** to increase the body's core temperature. It takes around ten minutes for the body to warm up and athletes can use light jog or bike spin to gradually raise their heart rate from Zone 1 to Zone 2. Full-body movements like jumping jacks, skipping rope, among others, can be used to achieve the same effect.

- **Muscle activation exercises and form drills** to "turn on" relevant muscles that are required for correct and efficient form. To activate mind-muscle connection, in a way. This is typically achieved with muscle-isolation exercises using resistance bands (light pressure, slow execution to feel the relevant muscles engaging) and very short speed and technique drills (done explosively or at the desired workout effort). A soft foam roller (1–2 rolls only) or a massage gun can also be used to help activate the muscles.

COOL DOWN AND MUSCLE RELEASE

Fatigue and muscle tightness build up over time and actions that athletes take immediately following a training practice can have a direct effect on that. In particular, light movement and muscle release activities stimulate utilization of fatigue and speeds up muscle recovery, which is why athletes should give themselves time after practice before jumping to other daily commitments. Otherwise, their muscles will require more time to fully recover. A "cool down" acts as a transition period that helps the body and mind relax after an intense practice and switch from workout mode to normal.

As little as 10 minutes of low-intensity activity speeds up the process of clearing the lactate and other metabolic waste from the muscles. Oxygen and other nutrients get to the muscles faster. Toxins also get eliminated quicker. Levels of adrenaline and cortisol are lower and the nervous system is able to relax and use the energy to rebuild torn tissues. All of it makes adaptations happen sooner and promotes better and more sustainable fitness gains. On top of that, it is important to do a form of muscle release after a training practice (or generally in the evening) to return muscles to their normal length, relieve muscle tightness and promote blood flow.

- **Deep stretching:** At least a full minute of stretch time in each position done until slight discomfort and with deep breathing.
- **Foam rolling:** Five to six targeted rolls per muscle group (medium to hard roller). No need to spend half a day on a roller.
- **Massage:** A full hour session once every week or two. Alternatively, ten minutes of self-massage or on an acupressure mat after every high intensity session.

SNEAK PEEK: TRIGGER POINT THERAPY TO RELIEVE MUSCLE TIGHTNESS

2010 was shaping up to be my best season in kayaking. Even before the season began, I had already logged in hundreds of hours of running, cross country skiing and kayaking, as well as leveled up my strength training routine. My form was good and at spring training camp, I was way ahead of my past year's splits at every control. Things were looking promising.

However, a month after returning from that training camp I started to feel weak. As if all of the power and endurance I had built until that point was suddenly taken out. Lifting my arms became a struggle, I couldn't breathe in fully and was getting tired quickly during training practice and throughout the day. My body was aching in various places for no particular reason and even after recovery sessions. It was frustrating and scary, especially since every doctor I visited told me everything was fine. On paper, I was at my best. Every test came out perfect and confirmed my health was good. Internally, though, I felt miserable. Something was way off.

During a VO_2max test I explained my situation to a sports physician. She also couldn't tell what it was that made me feel so strange but asked a physiotherapist to take a look. What happened next was the breakthrough in my body and mind. Within a few minutes that physiotherapist moved my arms and torso into certain positions that made bones in my body make a few cracking sounds. I felt an instant relief, as if I dropped a heavy backpack I was carrying. Breathing got easier and I felt a sense of ease and lightness despite having gone to the limit in the VO_2max test just an hour earlier.

What that physiotherapist did was use trigger point therapy to release tightness in my chest. With the increase in volume and pressure came a lot of tension, so the harder I trained the tighter the body got. My muscles were so locked up that I was stuck in a limbo: not able to push hard to improve, but also not recovering well. Obviously, one such therapy didn't solve the issue entirely, but that was a major lesson for me to focus more on muscle release in between training sessions. Going forward, I noticed that whenever I achieved a certain range of motion in my muscles, whatever discomfort I had experienced vanished, and I was able to deliver better performance.

CORE AND MOBILITY TRAINING

Intense training schedule and/or sedentary lifestyles can leave our muscles tight and inefficient. **More often than not, such common issues like knee and lower back pain can be attributed to the weakness of certain supporting muscles.** Mobility work includes rehabilitation exercises that make those small but very important areas stronger. It uses a combination of stretches and functional movements to replicate a desired pattern. To an athlete who performs at the top of his or her abilities, these exercises might not look sexy. Nor does it feel impressive to use resistance bands and the smallest dumbbells in the gym when you are used to lifting big weights. However, working on weak areas in such a way ultimately allows an athlete to produce more powerful and coordinated movements that make all the difference in the sport.

A strong core complements mobility. It is a group of muscles located in the center of the body and acts as a central hub (hence the name) that keeps all adjacent muscles aligned and healthy. All muscles that attach to the spine contribute to a strong core, abs, lower back, obliques, hips, glutes, adductors, and even lats. They help to distribute the load effectively across the body to those muscle groups that are designed best for the purpose, and also to ensure no muscle or joint is tight or unable to operate. Essentially, the core connects the upper and lower body and provides stability and control over all body movements, which, among other things, improves performance, promotes good posture and reduces the risk of many injuries.

Effective core and mobility training requires two things: good form and time under tension. Forget about weights and repetitions, it is better to do a little but correctly, at slow speed and with good form to engage the right muscles. Try to control the movement and avoid any shaking, rocking, or wiggling. Instead of doing complex movements right away, focus on building basic strength across the whole body first. Take your time to go from beginner exercises (bridges, planks) to advanced ones (side planks, exercises on unstable surfaces).

Get into the practice of doing a form of core and mobility work daily to keep the body aligned. Be it by joining a Yoga or Pilates class or as simple as doing a ten-minute core routine. As long as you are moving the body in every way every day, you are making it more resilient.

TRAIN WHERE YOU ARE

Planning is an important element of success and helps to set a trajectory for an athlete to improve. Personally, I thrive on planning my season and enjoy doing it for the athletes I coach. It feels deeply motivating to set lofty goals and sketch a route to reach them. However, throughout the season, and life for that matter, it is rare that everything goes exactly as intended. Simon Sinek nailed the wisdom when he said, "Always plan for the fact that no plan ever goes according to plan." We need to have a trajectory, but at the end of the day, all that really matters is where we are in the present moment and what the next step is going to be. So, while a plan, target or ambition is absolutely necessary, being flexible within that big picture is equally important.

A lot of athletes have a definite goal in mind, to qualify for Boston, complete an Ironman triathlon, or even one as cliche as losing a few pounds. Naturally, this creates certain expectations about the timeline (i.e., how quickly the goal can be achieved) and a desire to get there faster. However, most of the setbacks occur because athletes want to shortcut the process. Yes, it's possible to get fit very fast by putting the body through an enormous training load. But what's the point of it if the body breaks?

Whatever expectations for the race, fitness or health are, the body is our best guide. It has its own pace and we cannot enforce certain expectations on it. When we chase an artificial standard, an appearance, a time goal or even a feeling, we get emotionally attached to it and disconnected from reality—so much so that some actions might be detrimental to health and performance. Instead, we should work with the body to find the rate of improvement that it is comfortable with. Be realistic and train based on where your physical condition currently is, not where we want it to be.

Every person is on their own Hero's Journey. Some are at their peak fitness, while others are recovering from an injury. Some are young athletes who are just stepping up, whereas others are more senior and experienced. That's just the way it is. Everyone has their own agenda and the only person we should compare ourselves to is who we were yesterday.

> *Be you. It is not about measuring yourself against any other person or what you used to be. It's paramount you train where you are, not where you wish you were. Not even where you hope you are, and definitely not where you think you should be.*

Too often, when we want to create change for ourselves, we feel the urge to do something radical: quit the job, move to a new city, end the relationship, or start a very intense training program. However, such bold moves require monumental effort and produce a lot of stress that's usually unmanageable in the long term.

The truth is, there is no elevator to where we want to get. So, we have to be honest with ourselves and take the stairs, which implies starting where we are right now. For example, if running is too difficult for you, find something else. Hiking, rucking, rowing, cycling, there are plenty of low impact activities to engage in. Whatever you do, always focus on getting a little bit stronger, going a little bit further and growing a little bit more. Even if it is by as little as a few percent. Such a change is much easier to handle on a frequent basis, and over time it will grow into a substantial shift that, most importantly, stays with you.

As much as resilience involves "bouncing back" from difficult experiences, it also entails profound personal growth. As we learned through this book, it is not a trait that people either have or do not have. It implies thoughts, actions and behaviors that can be learned and developed by anyone.

Anyone can build the foundation of health and fitness that an athlete can rely on throughout his or her life. Doing the "maintenance work" to avoid an issue or an injury getting in the way of living life (i.e., a bad knee or back pain). And in the unfortunate case of injury or other complications that prevent an athlete from following his or her passion, refocusing energy and mindset towards reinvention, embracing the beginner's mindset and thinking, '*How can I put myself in the best position for growth?*'

As you've witnessed throughout this book, there is a lot that goes into producing top performance. Showing up at 100% and realizing his or her full potential requires an athlete to put equal effort in developing a strong mindset, cultivating habits that energize and using effective training techniques. When an athlete looks at his or her life from such a holistic perspective, training becomes the lifestyle. That focus on the long term and consistent reinvention across all aspects of performance is what makes an athlete truly resilient.

EXERCISE: REINVENT YOURSELF

If you watch closely how children (5+ years) run on the playground, you might notice a lot of similarities with elite runners. They have good arm action and a slight forward lean. Their body is aligned, they land under their center of mass and with every swing of the leg, their foot travels far back before quickly coming very close to their backside, and their movements are so fluid that it's a joy to watch. Kids do that naturally; nobody really taught them how to run. Add some endurance to such form and you will get a great runner. Most of the hobby runners, however, barely lift their legs from the ground, are hunched forward, and generally look very tight. Because they are and functional mobility is one of the reasons why there are so many talented athletes in college, but very few make it further.

When one part of the body becomes tight, it can compromise the entire structural alignment. In particular, it will force the load on larger muscles to compensate, thereby weakening the stabilizing muscles and reducing the range of motion. It amplifies over hundreds of hours of training and daily activities, prevents our body from operating efficiently, and can even lead to injuries. By addressing such imbalance and mobility blocks, athletes can not only reverse some of their chronic pains, but also open up a lot of extra performance capacity.

For this exercise, I ask you to apply your skill of personal detective and note some of the discomforts and chronic pains you experience, whether lately or in general. Consult with a qualified physical therapist to understand what causes the pain and holds you back, as well as research the possible ways of reversing the condition. Once you discover an area of weakness, use the heal-release-strengthen method to address the root of the problem instead of just treating the symptoms:

1.   **If you are in pain, stop training and regroup.** Take a few weeks off from exercise and let the joint or muscle heal fully. No challenge, adventure or race is worth sacrificing health for. Pushing through the pain will not make it go away and will only increase the risk of developing a chronic condition.

2.   **Once the pain subsides, focus on increasing your range of motion across the entire body.** Start with major muscle groups (legs, back, chest) and use deep stretching and foam rolling on a daily basis to release muscle tightness.

3.   **Start rebuilding strength from the ground up.** Go back to the basics and address structural issues. Use bodyweight and simple exercises, and don't rush to increase the load. Perform the repetitions slowly and be aware of every movement to ensure that even the smallest muscles are activated. The more control you gain over the body, the more balanced and aligned it becomes.

Keep investigating and seeking ways to constantly reinvent yourself. Resilient athletes have the courage to slow down or even start again. But when they do so, it is for the purpose of going even further.

AFTERWORD: LIFE IS AN ADVENTURE

"It ain't about how hard ya hit. It's about how hard you can get it and keep moving forward. How much you can take and keep moving forward. That's how winning is done!"

— ROCKY BALBOA

When you are in the flow or otherwise fully immersed in an activity, you never focus on things that can go wrong. Such thoughts can break the focus and limit the capacity to go beyond the comfort zone that is paramount to producing your best performance. As an athlete, by virtue of hundreds of hours spent challenging yourself to get stronger, you learn to become virtually bulletproof in your mind and your body. However, not thinking about a potential accident does not mean it cannot catch you off guard, and that is when the awakening comes.

An athlete's life is filled with tales of great victories, personal records, or individual triumphs. But there are also defeats, struggles, and experiences that one would rather forget. The story ahead is one of those kinds.

My first triathlon race didn't go exactly as planned, to say the least. I had never raced a bike in competition and didn't know what to expect from an individual start. In my head, since it was only 40K (~25mi) I tried to bike hard and catch up with whoever was in front of me. Basically, how most of my kayaking events in the past unfolded. The concept of keeping it easy, conserving energy and saving something for the run was removed from my memory that day. At the halfway mark, there was one particularly long descent with smooth turns. A thought went through my mind: '*Shouldn't my hands be on the brakes while descending at 70 km/h?'* I repositioned my hands from aero position to brakes and back several times. I really had no clear idea what I was doing at that moment but focused on pushing hard. Fueled by excitement, I powered over the hill only to notice another descent in front of me. This time, though, it was sharp and went through a cute German village with small houses and neat driveways pinched closely together. The visibility was very impaired, as the road zigzagged its way down. Gaining speed, I got distracted trying to figure out which direction the road would go and spotted the *Slow!* markings on the road a little too late. Noticing that I was quickly approaching the side of the road, my left hand reached for the front brake, while my right hand stayed on the aero bars to keep balance.

I don't recall the moment of impact. Somehow my tired, dehydrated, and oblivious mind decided not to store the memory of that. Instead, the very next thing I remember was lying on the side of the road, staring at a concrete wall in front of me with my right leg still clipped to the bike. What happened was that I hit a curb at 50km/h, flew over the handlebars, went down on my hip, "brushed" someone's driveway for several meters and stopped just a few centimeters away from a concrete wall. Had there been a car parked, it would have gone much worse.

I checked my helmet—no signs of cracks. Good, it seems that I didn't hit my head. Now arms and legs. A couple of hard bruises on the hip and elbow, but everything seemed to move without too much pain. Another good sign. Next was the bike , and from the looks of it, the wheel took the hardest hit and got crooked in such a way that it was facing 45 degrees to the left from the handlebars. Riding further was not an option. As I was inspecting my bike and figuring out how in the world I would get to the transition area, a red cross volunteer appeared beside me. By that time, I had gotten past the initial shock reaction and the pain in my hip and elbow started to grow. The volunteer helped me hobble down to the bottom of the descent where the medical tent was, so that I could sit down and get inspected. The descent ended with a sharp 90-degree left turn, which was not in sight in the place where I crashed. Honestly, I couldn't imagine how I would have maneuvered that turn in the position I was in had I not crashed.

In the meantime, volunteers were spending quite a lot of time inspecting my elbow and repeating in German, "Fraktur, fraktur." I was surprised that they were not paying any attention to the hip, which—obvious to me—was hurting much more. What was wrong with my elbow? Slowly, feelings and a sense of reality started coming back to me. As I was leaving the "beast mode" I started feeling thirsty. In fact, I was so dehydrated that my head started to turn and I lost balance. Seeing me in such a state, even though I was fully aware of what was happening, the medics told me my race was over. It felt strange and scary at the same time. While I did have some DNFs in my kayaking career, I was never in a situation when someone told me I could not continue.

I signed up for this race at the last minute to get some practice before what I thought would be the highlight of my season—the Half Ironman triathlon taking place 2 weeks later. The intention behind a shorter race was to remain in Zone 3 to simulate the intensity I would need to maintain, as well as practice nutrition, transitions, logistics, and small practicalities. It was a good plan. Too bad I didn't stick to it.

I feel that crash was life's way of intervening to make me stop and reconsider my purpose. It had done its job: driving home all bruised and bandaged, certain thoughts were circling in my head. Will I be OK? Could I ride a steep hill on a bike again? Am I my best self? Is it sustainable? I realized that I was in this situation before. Feeling down—emotionally and physically—and not knowing whether I can or should go on. I remembered that cold morning in the middle of rural Latvia. Halfway through the overnight kayak marathon when I was on the verge of giving up, exhausted, cold, and hungry at the same time, but I got through it. So, I knew I would get through this as well. Hard patches come up, but eventually pass. I have come a long way since that night and every experience I had helped set myself up for this day. I just needed to pick myself up, dust off, adjust the course a little and, most importantly, get going.

At the core of every Hero's Journey is a desire to step into the unknown, seek adventure, and above all, embrace reinvention. Everyone told me I was crazy to race again two weeks after a crash. But then again, nobody knew about the transformation that was taking place. All of the gradual changes I made to my training and lifestyle so far, got me in the best physical shape of my life, even better than when I trained for the European and World Championships. That DNF was an opportunity to take it even further. As painful as the experience was, it served its purpose and made me more resilient. It reminded me that we can never have everything figured out. Even when we think we do, things change. So, there is always time for reinvention, always time to do more and grow stronger. Coming to the sport of triathlon I believed I was a strong athlete but was quickly reminded of how much there is still left to work on.

As I was standing on the start line just two weeks following the crash, I was in a totally different mindset. The race wasn't this tough ordeal anymore and I wasn't there to chase any results. Instead, it felt like a celebration of the journey that led me to the start line. I realized that when you remove expectations, you are truly living and, ironically, when you can fully focus on delivering your best performance. '*Could I have gone faster had I not had the crash? Would I be able to deliver an even better performance had I been more aggressive on technical parts of the course?*' I don't know, but I know these are not the right concerns to have. The only question that is worthy of answering is why? And for what purpose? For me, the entire journey of getting to that particular start line marked a major milestone in the process of profound transformation. I went from a professional kayaker to a runner to triathlete and, eventually, a coach.

Developing a growth mindset, optimizing the lifestyle to have more energy for the things that matter ad changing my training to be ready to take on any adventure, all of it helped me erase the limits and learn that by doing one small step (supercompensation) at a time that I was able to completely pivot my life towards a stronger, healthier and more self-actualized version of myself that I didn't think existed. I bring that quality and energy into everything I do and feel privileged to be able to share it with you.

ACKNOWLEDGEMENTS

Writing this book has been a Hero's Journey in and of itself for me. With all its elements—the call for adventure, finding mentors, overcoming personal challenges and, of course, emerging on the other side reborn and enlightened. I relived some of the brightest and lowest moments of my life and organized them in a healthy way. Yes, this process has put all of my knowledge and experience to the test, as I juggled writing, working a day job, being present for my family, training for a marathon and running a coaching business—all on a very tight timeline. I've put my heart and soul into this project and am very proud of the result.

It might seem I did all of it myself, but the reality is that none of the journeys happen in isolation. This book is no exception and wouldn't be possible without all of the support I have had along the way—intentional or not. And for that I would like to express my sincere gratitude.

To my wife for being my muse and the best support crew an athlete could wish for. You are always there for me—be it to dream big, help me not to lose sight of my vision when faced with a difficult situation or simply to hand me a missing gel at the later stage of a marathon. I wouldn't be where I am today without all the love, care and attention you have given me over the years.

To my parents for giving me the freedom to explore and experiment while being patient as I jumped from one sport to another trying to learn to control my energy. You taught me to always finish what I have started and never let go when things get tough. Developing that discipline didn't come easy to me and only now have I begun to appreciate the value of that backbone.

To my training partners whom I trained with during my professional kayaking career for always keeping me on my toes. We pushed each other to the limit during competitions, as well as during intense and long sessions. But we always made sure none of us were left behind. The best man at my wedding has expressed that brilliantly: "All those hours spent going through hard work together, they don't just go away. Instead, they create a special lasting bond."

To the many coaches I have had throughout my training career for teaching me the value of effort and consistent work. Having the opportunity to be exposed to different training methodologies gave me a broad perspective and helped to develop my own framework. Thank you all for believing in me, sharing your time, giving me guidance and mentoring along the way.

To the people at Hatherleigh Press who helped me find an angle in my experience and guided me in turning that into a shareable idea that became this book.